OXFORD MEDICAL PUBLICATIONS

Epilepsy

THE FACTS

ALSO PUBLISHED BY OXFORD UNIVERSITY PRESS

Epilepsy

THE FACTS
Second Edition

ANTHONY HOPKINS

Director, Research Unit,
Royal College of Physicians, London

and

RICHARD APPLETON

Department of Neurology,
Alder Hey Children's Hospital, Liverpool

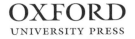

OXFORD
UNIVERSITY PRESS

OXFORD

UNIVERSITY PRESS

Great Clarendon Street, Oxford OX2 6DP

Oxford University Press is a department of the University of Oxford.
It furthers the University's objective of excellence in research, scholarship,
and education by publishing worldwide in

Oxford New York

Athens Auckland Bangkok Bogotá Buenos Aires Calcutta
Cape Town Chennai Dar es Salaam Delhi Florence Hong Kong Istanbul
Karachi Kuala Lumpur Madrid Melbourne Mexico City Mumbai
Nairobi Paris São Paulo Singapore Taipei Tokyo Toronto Warsaw

with associated companies in Berlin Ibadan

Oxford is a registered trade mark of Oxford University Press
in the UK and in certain other countries

Published in the United States
by Oxford University Press Inc., New York

First edition published in hardback in 1981 and in paperback in 1984
Second edition published 1996
Reprinted 1999

A catalogue record for this book is available from the British Library

Library of Congress Cataloging in Publication Data
Hopkins, Anthony.
Epilepsy / Anthony Hopkins and Richard Appleton.
p. cm.—(The Facts)
Previously published : Oxford : Oxford University Press, 1981.
Includes index.
ISBN 0 19 262548 9 (pbk)
1. Epilepsy—Popular works. I. Appleton, Richard. II. Title.
III. Series: Facts (Oxford, England)
RC372.H58 1995
616.8'53—dc20 95-39526
CIP

Printed in Great Britain on acid-free paper by
Biddles Ltd, Guildford and King's Lynn

Contents

Introduction

There are all sorts of problems about epilepsy, which we hope this small book will do something to dispel. Epilepsy is the name given to recurrent 'seizures' (also known as 'fits', or 'attacks'), of which the fairly well-known grand mal convulsions are only one type. A whole variety of brain disorders can cause epilepsy, which should perhaps be considered no more than a stereotyped reaction of the brain to a variety of stresses. It is not generally known that, in spite of the most modern methods of investigation, an underlying cause can only be identified with certainty in about one third of people with epilepsy. The good news that has emerged from research studies over the last twenty years is that the long-term outlook for the cessation of seizures is very much better than was previously considered to be the case, as earlier research referred only to people with epilepsy whose seizures were the most difficult to control.

People with epilepsy have many worries. Children with epilepsy may be upset or worried about telling their friends and what will happen to them in the future. Women with epilepsy are understandably concerned about the possible effects of anti-epileptic medication when pregnant. Not everyone understands the impact of epilepsy upon the eligibility to hold a driving licence. Many employers understand little about epilepsy, and people with epilepsy may not have the same possibilities of employment, or of career advancement. These are among the concerns which this book addresses.

As the figure on page 17 indicates, epilepsy can begin at any age in life, but is particularly likely to begin in early childhood. One of us is a paediatric neurologist with a particular interest in epilepsy, and the other works with adults with epilepsy. We hope that this book will be read by people with epilepsy, by their parents and relatives, and by members of the teaching, nursing, and social work professions who need a clear introduction to this troublesome disorder.

1 *What is epilepsy?*

How nerve cells work

The human brain contains about 100 000 million nerve cells, each of which is connected to many others—perhaps as many as 50 000 others. The brain is the organ of our thinking and of our memory. It integrates information from the outside world and so allows us to perceive objects and events around us. It organizes our response to these events by movements or other action. It organizes our social behaviour.

Messages are passed between nerve cells by the extraordinarily rapid secretion of tiny packets of specialized chemicals known as *neurotransmitters*. As a neurotransmitter acts on the next cell in a chain, a brief electric current is generated. These can be recorded by very fine wires placed next to or in a nerve cell, but they are not large enough to be recorded externally over the skin of the head. However, some cells act in rhythmic concert, and these rhythms can be detected as the *electroencephalogram* (EEG) over the skin of the hands by small electrodes amplified, recorded on tape or disc, and displayed on a moving strip of paper or screen. The use of this procedure is described in Chapter 5.

Some messages received by a nerve cell are inhibitory—they dampen down the activity of the receiving cell; some are excitatory, enhancing its activity. The receiving nerve cell computes, as it were, these contrasting messages, which determine its own action.

The events leading to a seizure

One of the ways in which events can go wrong is when a nerve cell loses some of its inputs from other cells because of damage to these other nerve cells. If inhibitory terminals are lost, then the cell will become over-excitable, and begin to switch on, or fire inappropriately, driving other nerve cells with which it is connected on the downstream side to similar activity. This may result in more and more nerve cells being incorporated into the abnormal pattern of discharge.

The biological background of an epileptic seizure is therefore an abnormal discharge of nerve cells in the cerebral hemispheres of the brain. The normal, quiet, and integrated function of nerve cells is interrupted as they are forced through the contacts they make with and receive from others into a paroxysmal discharge. Different types of seizure are a reflection of different patterns of paroxysmal discharge. Seizure types are described in Chapter 2 and two examples will suffice here. If the seizure discharge spreads throughout large areas of the brain, then consciousness may be lost. If the discharge of nerve cells is confined to the temporal lobe of the brain (more or less above and in front of the ears), amongst those cells concerned with memory, the paroxysmal discharge may result only in a distortion of memory so that the sufferer perceives that he or she has experienced ongoing events before—the phenomenon of *déjà vu*.

The definition of an epileptic seizure

In someone with established epilepsy, the EEG between seizures may also show abnormal discharges which are not apparent to the doctor in terms of observed behaviour, nor are they associated with any change perceived by the person with epilepsy. Although the abnormal discharges of the EEG are clearly a fragment, as it were, of a seizure, they are not usually regarded as seizures. Our definition of an epileptic seizure, therefore, is a *paroxysmal discharge of cerebral nerve cells apparent to the person and/or an observer.*

Anything which increases the excitability of a group of nerve cells may cause a paroxysmal discharge. For example certain gases or chemicals, developed for use in war, are designed to cause disabling seizures amongst the enemy.

The definition of epilepsy

Although we hope that such gases will never be used, we have deliberately introduced the topic at this point to explain the difference between the diagnosis of *'an epileptic seizure'* and the diagnosis of *'epilepsy'*. It would clearly be ridiculous to label as 'epileptics' those soldiers who had convulsed on exposure to the nerve gas. The cause of their seizures is readily apparent, and, not only that, the tendency to convulse is present only in the presence of the nerve gas. Someone is said to suffer from *epilepsy* if he or she has a *continuing tendency to epileptic seizures.*

This example polarizes, as it were, the explanation, but there are many grey areas, some of which we explain here, and others will become apparent elsewhere in this book. Take for example the case of a young man who has a single seizure at the age of 19, after a rather-too-good office party at Christmas time. It would be justifiable to assume that alcohol played some part in the genesis of the seizure—but there were others who drank just as much who did not have a seizure. So we must presume that the man has a lower *convulsive threshold* than his colleagues (see p. 29). A single seizure is not considered sufficient to make the diagnosis of epilepsy, as, until time has passed, it will not be known whether or not this seizure will prove to be the first of others. However, as is discussed further on p. 81, about three-quarters of all such people will have a second seizure within three years.

Doctors will make a diagnosis of epilepsy when they hear of *more than one seizure of any type* not associated with fever. *Convulsions* associated with illness (febrile convulsions are discussed in Chapter 9). Clearly there is no difficulty in doing this if the time scale is short, but what do we call a man who has one fit at the age of 19 and another at the age of 80? It would seem a bit nonsensical to tell the elderly man that he had been an epileptic all his life, as we would be obliged to do if we followed rigidly the definition of 'more than one non-febrile seizure'. Another problem—what do we call a woman aged 40, who has had ten seizures between the ages of 15 and 25? We cannot, unfortunately, say that she is a 'woman cured of epilepsy', as experience shows she is still slightly at risk from further seizures (see p. 5). These examples clearly show that the label 'epilepsy' has to be applied with common sense. It is not one of those tidy diseases such as myocardial infarction, in which there is little argument about the heart attack or the coronary disease causing it.

These medical uncertainties are reflected in patients' minds. After all, if a doctor cannot give a crystal-clear definition of a disease, how can the patient be expected to understand it? The uncertainties in peoples' minds are compounded by a series of half-or un-truths that, perhaps because epilepsy is so common, are held in the collective imagination as folk lore—that epilepsy is inherited; that it begins in childhood; that it is always convulsive in nature; and that it is related in some ways to mental illness. Glimpses of this stereotype of epilepsy are seen in the clinic when a patient, or his relative, says 'it can't be epilepsy because . . . .' We hope that this book will dispel some of these confusions.

Part of the difficulty in understanding about epilepsy is a hangover from the ideas of the great physicians of the nineteenth century. 'Diseases' were described—for example, Bright's disease of the kidneys. Such diseases have proved unexpectedly more and more complex with further research. For example, Bright described the dilute urine containing protein, and changes associated with high blood pressure that are merely symptoms common to a number of processes resulting in chronic kidney failure.

With these comments in mind, an epileptic seizure should be regarded as a *symptom* —an event that is just one of the few ways that the brain has of reacting to untoward internal processes. The continuation of such reactions constitutes epilepsy. As to the causes of epilepsy, considered at length in Chapter 3, it is the doctor's task to disentangle, if at all possible, the factors that result in seizures.

We have had some difficulty in deciding what to call the child or person with epilepsy throughout this book. There are some who instinctively dislike the word—or label—'epileptic'. It is of course an adjective, and one does not talk about those with heart disease or multiple sclerosis as 'cardiacs' or 'multiple sclerotics'. We admit, however, that those with diabetes seem quite happy to be known as 'diabetics'. We find the word person too *im*personal, but to write and read 'a man, woman, or child with epilepsy' takes too long, and to write each time 'those with epilepsy' seems archaic. We have avoided the use of the word patient, except in a medical context, as people with epilepsy should only become patients for brief moments in their lives. We therefore use whatever phrase seems most appropriate in the context.

Words used to describe epileptic seizures

What about the words used to describe epileptic seizures? The word *'seizure'* is that most commonly used by neurologists for all types, but, depending upon the manifestation of the seizure, they may call them *convulsions*. Often they will use the words employed by their patients—for example, *fit, turn, attack or dizzy spell*. People who have two types of seizure often call them *'big ones'* and *'little ones'*. As long as the patient and the doctor find themselves talking about the same events, this is perfectly acceptable.

The word seizure is really too sudden and violent a word to describe the minor distortions of consciousness that may be the only manifestation of some types of epilepsy such as *absences*, but we do not have a better word to cover all types. We use it throughout in this book, with the exception of the section on febrile convulsions, a term hallowed by long usage, and, in any event, as we show in Chapter 9, only distantly related to epilepsy.

Sometimes in correspondence and conversation doctors employ the words *'epileptiform'* or *'epileptoid'*. In our experience, doctors who use such terms are skating round the subject and avoiding frankly stating that their patient has had an epileptic seizure. The only justification for such a term might be the description of attacks called *anoxic seizures* in which a few jerks of the limbs arise during a profound faint, in which the blood supply to the brain is briefly insufficient. Apart from this example, and strokes, which used to be called apoplectic seizures, by common usage in English-speaking countries a seizure now means an epileptic event.

How common is epilepsy?

The *incidence* of a disease means the number of *new* cases in a defined population (usually 100 000) in a defined period of time (usually one year).

Good figures for the incidence of new cases of epilepsy come from the population of Olmstead County in Minnesota. People in this

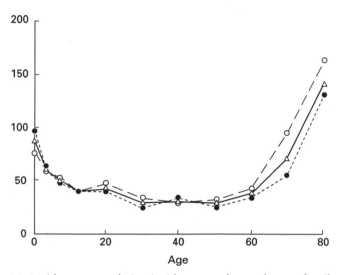

Fig. 1.1 Incidence, cumulative incidence, and prevalence of epilepsy at various ages. Vertical axis shows new cases per 100 000 per year. (Redrawn from Olmstead County study by kind permission of Dr A. Hauser.)

rural part of the USA do not move around very much, and have the good fortune to be cared for by doctors at the famous Mayo Clinic. Research workers there have long had an interest in identifying all patients with epilepsy.

Figure 1 shows the incidence of new cases of epilepsy (more than one non-febrile seizure) per 100 000 per year plotted against age of onset. The incidence of new cases is highest in infancy and in old age for reasons which are explained in Chapter 3, but new cases can occur at any age. Throughout middle life the incidence is about 40 cases per 100 000 per year. As the years go by, the risk of having had epilepsy at some time in one's life increases in a cumulative fashion. The cumulative incidence in a population of children studied in the UK was 410 per 100 000 by the age of eleven, 600 by the age of 16, and 1000 per 100 000 by the age of 23. From the United States study cited above, the cumulative risk by age 75 was 3400 per 100 000 (3.4 per cent) for males and 2800 per 100 000 (2.8 per cent) for females. Epilepsy is thus not a rare or unusual disorder; seizures may impinge upon the lives of any one of us.

Another word used in counting cases of disease is *prevalence*. Here it is best to consider first another common illness which has a prolonged and steady course such as Parkinson's disease. It is quite easy (though expensive) to do a door to door survey and count the people found to have Parkinson's disease, as the signs of it will always be apparent. Prevalence is usually expressed per 1000. The prevalence of cases per 1000 population means that this number of people have the disease on the day of the survey. This technique is more difficult for epilepsy because of its episodic nature. Clearly, common sense dictates that if someone had a seizure during a day on which a survey day was done, they should be included, but what about someone who had many seizures in the past, but none for three years? One has to judge where to draw the line. In practice, most surveys of prevalence include people who have had more than one non-febrile seizure in the past, and are on continuing anti-epileptic drugs and/or who have had at least one seizure in the last two years. After early childhood, the prevalence is more or less constant throughout life at about seven per 1000 in developed countries, and considerably higher in developing countries.

Does epilepsy stop?

There is one encouraging point that all those with epilepsy must remember—the number of people who have epilepsy at any one time is much less than those who have had epilepsy in the past. An approximate estimate of the *average* duration of epilepsy can be obtained by dividing the average prevalence by the average annual incidence. This gives a figure of about 11 years. However artificial this figure may be, it underlines the point that epilepsy can and does usually stop. A great number of people with epilepsy fare better. The factors which allow some prediction of what is the likely course for any person with epilepsy are considered in Chapter 7.

2 The different types of epileptic seizure and of epilepsy syndromes

Figure 2.1 illustrates the two main classes of origin of seizure. In the top third of the figure, the hatched area indicates a number of nerve cells in the cortex (the name given to the layers of nerve cells on the surface of the brain) which are in some way abnormal, tending to discharge paroxysmally. They may drive other nerve cells to follow their abnormal patterns of discharge. The paths of influence of the discharging nerve cells are indicated by the arrows. As long as the discharge remains in one part of the brain, the seizure is said to be a *partial seizure* and its cause *location-related*. What happens during a partial seizure depends upon the exact site and pattern of discharge of abnormal nerve cells. Temporal lobe seizures as described on p. 16 are of this type. The features of these are described in more detail on pp. 14–17, along with those of other types of partial seizures.

The abnormal discharge may spread through the connections linking the two halves of the brain, or, by affecting poorly identified central collections of cells, initiate a generalized seizure discharge, in which case the seizure is said to be a *partial seizure with secondary generalization* (to a convulsive seizure—grand mal). These are also known as tonic–clonic seizures for reasons which are explained on p. 12). This process is shown in the middle third of Fig. 2.1.

The lower third of Fig. 2.1 illustrates the second main class of seizure. In this class of seizure, central collections of nerve cells are in some way abnormal in their behaviour—even though they may appear to be perfectly normal under the microscope. Because of their central position, and the direction and power of their transmissions, a seizure discharge generated within them spreads more or less simultaneously to all parts of the brain. Such a seizure is generalized at onset. Typical absences (p. 13) (often known as petit mal), and some grand mal seizures, are of this type.

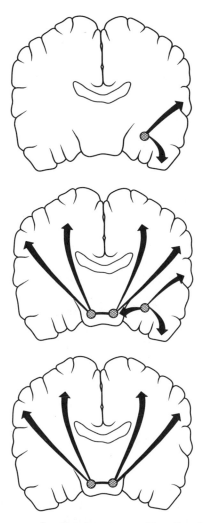

Fig. 2.1 Different types of epileptic seizure. *Top*: Partial seizure—the paroxysmal discharge spreads locally from a focus of abnormal cells in the cortex, here folded in in the temporal lobe. *Middle*: Partial seizure with secondary generalization—the discharge spreads locally, and also to centrally grouped nerve cells which spread the discharge widely through the brain. *Bottom*: Primary generalized seizure—the discharge spreads symmetrically throughout the brain from the beginning.

Grand mal seizures (tonic–clonic seizures)

Whether the paroxysmal discharge be primary, or secondarily generalized from a focus in the cortex, consciousness is lost if the seizure discharge involves much of the brain.

Cerebral nerve cells are connected to other nerve cells in the spinal cord. The powerful generalized cortical seizure discharge is therefore linked through this direct transmission system to muscle fibres. Disordered contraction of all muscles is the hallmark of a grand mal seizure.

The first phase of a grand mal seizure is known as the *tonic* (contraction) phase. At this stage, because of widespread contraction of muscles, the body is rigid, and is incapable of maintaining a normal coordinated posture, so that the person falls to the ground. The respiratory muscles also contract, forcing out the air in the chest, so there may be an involuntary noise—a grunt or a cry—at the onset of the attack. The jaw muscles also contract, and, because the normal associated movements that keep the tongue out of the way are disordered by the seizure discharge, the tongue or inside of the cheek may be bitten.

During the tonic phase there are no coordinated movements of breathing, yet muscular contraction caused by the seizure discharge is vigorous. This combination means that the oxygen in the blood is rapidly used up, and the subject will become a dusky blue colour, the technical name for which is cyanosis. This colour is exaggerated by dilatation of blood vessels in the face by raised pressure within the thorax, due to the strong contraction of chest muscles. Normal movements of swallowing are lost, so that saliva may dribble out between the tightly clenched teeth. The disordered contraction of abdominal and bladder muscles may result in incontinence of urine, though this is by no means invariable. Dilatation of the pupils and sweating often occur.

After one or two minutes of the tonic phase, the seizure passes into the *clonic* or convulsive phase, with rhythmic movements of limbs and trunk muscles. These gradually cease after a few minutes, and the child or adult lies passively unconscious, often breathing stertorously. Normal colour returns. Consciousness gradually lightens, so that they can be roused, then begin to move around, and then can be helped to their feet and a chair. For several minutes after this, they will be confused and restless. After this they may suffer a headache for the rest of the day, or go to bed and sleep for a couple of hours. They will also be aware of stiff and painful muscles which have contracted forcibly during the seizure.

Typical absences (petit mal seizures)

Although a translation of petit mal is the 'little illness', petit mal does not mean the same as 'minor epilepsy' as there are all sorts of small attacks which are *not* attacks of petit mal. True petit mal seizures, or typical absences are, by definition, associated with a characteristic EEG discharge, illustrated on p. 67. Short-lived partial seizures arising from a focus of abnormal nerve cells in one temporal lobe of the brain (see p. 16) may be somewhat similar on clinical grounds, but the distinction is worth making because of the difference in cause, treatment, and outcome between the two.

Absence epilepsy is virtually invariably a disorder of childhood. A typical attack is very brief, lasting only a few seconds. The onset and termination are abrupt. The child will suddenly cease what she is doing, stare, look a little pale, perhaps flutter her eyelids, and drop her head slightly forwards. Posture of the limbs and trunk is usually maintained so she does not fall. After the seizure, the child resumes what she has been doing. Because the interruption of the normal stream of consciousness is so brief, attacks may be unobserved by parents, and not remarked upon by the affected children. One of us has seen a typical attack in a supermarket. A girl aged about nine was helping her mother unload a wire basket at the checkout. She suddenly paused, with a pot of honey held in the air between basket and counter, fluttered her eyelids, and then continued transferring the purchase without further pause.

Whereas one would be unfortunate to have more then one grand mal seizure in a day, absence seizures may be very frequent—10 to 50 seizures a day being occasionally encountered. Fortunately most children have far fewer attacks.

Absence seizures are often associated with *myoclonic jerks*, which are particularly frequent soon after waking. These are brief shock-like contractions of the muscles, which are so short-lived it is not really possible to tell whether consciousness is disturbed or not. We have heard this described by one family as 'the flying saucer syndrome' in reference to the broken crockery that may occur as a result of jerks at breakfast-time!

Partial seizures

The exact internal perception or external manifestations of partial seizures depend upon the site of origin of discharge of abnormal nerve cells. If these lie in the part of the brain called the motor cortex, a strip of brain concerned with movement (Fig. 2.2), the initial manifestation will be a contraction of muscles in the opposite side of the body, as, through evolutionary events that are not entirely clear, one side of the brain controls the opposite side of the body. Cells in the motor cortex which supply the index finger and thumb, the corner of the mouth, or the big toe are most likely to be those in which a seizure discharge begins. There are more cells assigned to controlling these muscles, which are concerned with the fine tuning of manual skills and facial expression. Statistically, therefore, there is a greater chance of abnormal events occurring in these cells, but also experiments show that they are particularly easy to excite. The first evidence of such a partial seizure may be twitching of one corner of the mouth. As the seizure discharge spreads, the muscles around the eyes are next involved, as nerve cells supplying these muscles are next door to those supplying the mouth. Next involved are the hand muscles, and next the foot muscles. This march of events was described in the last century independently by Bravais, a French neurologist, and by Hughlings Jackson, an English neurologist whose wife had such attacks. This type of seizure is therefore often called a *Jacksonian seizure*. It may occur with no disturbance of consciousness whatsoever, as the discharge remains confined to the motor cortex. Partial seizures in which there is no disturbance of consciousness are said to be *simple partial seizures*.

Another type of partial seizure with movement is known as a *versive (turning) seizure*. In this the head and eyes turn to one side.

Usually the arm on the side to which they are turned is elevated and twitches. Sometimes the 'version' may continue so that the subject turns round several times on his own axis. Version is usually in the direction away from the discharging cerebral nerve cells—a left hemisphere focus causes turning to the right. Such seizures are therefore called *adversive*.

In the types of seizure described so far, there is an external manifestation—contraction of muscles driven by the discharging cerebral nerve cells, so that this type of seizure is easily apparent to an observer.

Most people are right handed, the left hemisphere then being considered to be *dominant*. Language is very largely located in the dominant hemisphere. An *aphasic partial seizure* in which expression or comprehension of language is impaired may arise from a seizure discharge in the dominant temporal lobe.

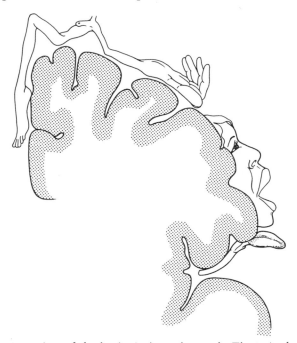

Fig. 2.2 A section of the brain (orientation as in Fig 2.1), showing the motor cortex and a drawing of the parts of the body controlled by different areas (after Penfield).

Other groups of discharging cerebral nerve cells may not necessarily result in any external apparent event, only in a distorted internal perception. A focus in one parietal lobe (just behind the motor cortex) may only result in a transient disturbance of sensation, such as a perception of pins and needles in the opposite side of the face, arm, or leg. A seizure discharge in the anterior part of one temporal lobe may result only in the person perceiving a strange smell, unreal, often unpleasant, and yet often vaguely familiar. Similar hallucinations of distorted taste may also occur, which are usually perceived as unpleasant.

If the seizure discharge begins in a slightly different part of the temporal lobe, complex visual hallucinations may occur. A boy of 11 told one of us that he saw himself standing near a shower with another boy, whom he felt he knew yet could not name. This boy and he alternately put their feet under the running water, and this odd hallucination continued until the seizure ended.

Other seizures arising in the temporal lobe may cause a perception that events taking place have previously occurred in the person's experience. This phenomenon is known as '*déjà vu*'. *Jamais vu* is a phrase used to indicate that the person perceives familiar surroundings as unreal.

If such distorted perceptions occur they may disturb full consciousness—as defined by awareness of current events, interpretation of current events, and correct responsiveness to current events. All gradations of disturbance of consciousness may be seen. For example, the child or adult may respond appropriately to a question after a considerable delay, or he may respond inappropriately, or not at all. After the attack has terminated, people may say that they were dimly aware of ongoing real events, but this is not necessarily true, and the person may have no memory for all events during and for some time after the seizure. Partial seizures in which consciousness is disturbed are said to be *complex partial seizures*.

Sometimes seizures arising in the temporal lobe result in complex automatic behaviour —a so-called *psychomotor seizure*. The person may, for example, dress and undress repeatedly or drum his fingers on the table. Less complex, but more common manifestations, are repeated sucking or chewing or swallowing movements. The person will have no memory for these events after the attack.

Such automatic behaviour occurring during the seizure discharge must be distinguished from the common confusion following a grand mal attack, or following a prolonged temporal lobe seizure, for which the person will also be amnesic. This amnesia is, perhaps, analogous of the amnesia following a head injury, in which, for example, a young man will complete a game of rugby football after a collision resulting in a concussive head injury, yet afterwards he will be amnesic for this part of the game.

Emotional experiences are very frequent in partial seizures arising in the temporal lobe. These are often expressed just as 'a horrible feeling', but sometimes the sensation of fear is overpowering.

Sensations in the abdomen and chest often also occur. A common initial sensation is a vague feeling of discomfort in the upper abdomen, which rises rapidly into the chest and head. The abdominal sensation may be accompanied by contractions of the stomach and bowel resulting in audible rumbles.

Another frequent internal sensation is one of vertigo. People with seizures beginning in the temporal lobe may say that they are 'dizzy.' This word is used in different senses by various people, but some appear to perceive vertigo (a sense of dysequilibrium which may be rotational) as part of the seizure.

Any partial seizure may become secondarily generalized into a tonic–clonic seizure (grand mal seizure) (see Figure 2.1). Sometimes this happens so quickly that the partial (focal) onset is only apparent on careful analysis of an EEG recorded during a seizure.

Rarer types of seizure

Atypical absences (petit mal variant)

This phrase is used in two different ways—to describe absences which are clinically similar to typical absences associated with an EEG record that is not typical, and to describe absences in association with other features which are not typical, of which loss of postural control is the most marked. In these fortunately unusual so-called 'akinetic drop attacks', children may crash to the floor with such force and frequency that they have to wear a crash helmet to protect the head from damage.

Clonic seizures

The distinction between these and myoclonic jerks (p. 13) is slight.
If jerks are multiple, then the seizures tend to be called clonic.

Tonic seizures

A tonic (rigid) posturing of all limbs without a clonic phase is sometimes seen in some generalized cerebral disorders in childhood. The
same name is given to one rare form of partial seizure in which one
part of the body briefly maintained abnormal tonic posture. Such
seizures may occasionally occur in adults with multiple sclerosis.

Infantile spasms (salaam seizures; West's syndrome)

These seizures of infancy are characterized by a brief, sudden flexion
of head, trunk, and limbs, as if the baby is bowing a 'salaam.' The
infant may appear to be thrown forwards or backwards with the
arms outstretched. Each spasm lasts about one second or less. The
spasms may occur in runs or clusters (up to 40–50 spasms per
cluster) over a 5–10 minute period; when this happens the infant
may appear distressed afterwards and cry. Spasms are more likely
to occur at certain times of the day, either just after the infant
has woken up from a sleep, or is about to fall asleep. In some
children, the spasms may occur almost continuously throughout
the day, happening several times an hour. The EEG in infants with
this type of seizure shows very abnormal patterns of activity called
hypsarrhythmia (see Fig. 5.5 in Chapter 5).

Further definitions

There are a few more aspects of epileptic seizures that require
explanation.

Some people may have a warning of seizure. The first type of
warning is a vague feeling of an impending seizure, particularly

before a tonic–clonic (grand mal) seizure. This *prodrome* may last several hours. It has no obvious physiological explanation, but it is remarked upon too often by people to be lightly dismissed as due to imaginary reconstruction of events. The prodrome is usually unpleasant—a feeling of mental heaviness or depression. Less commonly, elation and energetic activity may herald a seizure. The second type of warning, known as an *aura*, is not really a warning at all, but the initial symptom of the seizure itself. Examples of such auras include the epigastric sensation of partial seizures arising in one part of the temporal lobe, or the brief tingling in one hand which precedes a partial seizure arising in the parietal lobe which rapidly generalizes to a grand mal seizure.

Another phrase requiring definition is *post-ictal paresis*. An *ictus* is another older synonym for a seizure. Post-ictal paresis indicates weakness of left or right limbs following a convulsion primarily affecting those limbs. Sometimes known as Todd's paresis, after the neurologist who first described it, it indicates some structural problem in the hemisphere on the side opposite to the weak limbs. The weakness may last from a few minutes up to 48 hours. Post-ictal amnesia, post-ictal confusion, post-ictal sleep, and post-ictal headache have already been described. *Post-ictal automatism* is the phenomenon in which a person can undertake some fairly complex act, such as undressing and putting themselves to bed, of which they have no subsequent memory. *Status epilepticus* is a phrase used to indicate seizures occurring so close together that one seizure runs into another, without recovery of normal cerebral function between seizures. This may happen with any type of seizure, so that a neurologist speaks of absence status, partial status, or tonic–clonic (grand mal) status. In the first two types, the diagnosis may be difficult to reach unless the subject is already known to the doctor. The person may be found in the street or at home confused and inaccessible to conversation because of continuing seizure discharges (pp. 103–5).

Grand mal status epilepticus, in which the person does not recover consciousness between generalized tonic–clonic convulsions, is a medical emergency. The lack of normal respiratory movements, in association with the extreme muscular contractions during the seizures, throw a considerable stress upon the cardiovascular system. The principles of treatment of this serious but fortunately uncommon state are discussed on pp. 105–6, but early admission to hospital is essential.

Finally, a partial seizure in which the seizure discharge continues but remains confined to one part of the motor cortex results in continuous twitching of muscles in one part of a limb on the opposite side of the body. For example, the index finger and thumb may continue to twitch for days or even weeks, without any spread of seizure discharge to other muscles, and with no disturbance of consciousness. This is known as *epilepsia partialis continua*.

Epilepsy syndromes

So far we have considered the principal different types of epileptic seizures.

Paediatricians and neurologists recognize that certain clusters of symptoms and signs and patients' characteristics go together, and this is what we mean by a syndrome. The idea of epilepsy syndromes goes back many years, but a revised scheme or classification of epilepsy was proposed by the International League Against Epilepsy (ILAE) in 1989. In this classification, an epileptic syndrome is characterized by both clinical and EEG findings. On the clinical side, the age at onset of seizures, the family history, the seizure type(s), and neurological findings are all relevant to the classification, as is the appearance of the EEG between and during seizures. Identifying epileptic syndromes allows greater precision of diagnosis and of prognosis than simply classifying seizure types.

The same type of seizure can occur in different syndromes. For example, tonic–clonic (grand mal) seizures can occur in association with typical absences (primary generalized epilepsy in Fig. 2.3) or in association with partial seizures (location-related epilepsy). Conversely a person with one syndrome may have seizures of more than one type. For example, a child with primary generalized epilepsy may have both absence and tonic–clonic seizures (both petit and grand mal). Identifying an epileptic syndrome helps to select the most appropriate investigations, decide on the most appropriate

Table 2.1 Epilepsy syndromes classified by age of onset

Newborn period	Benign familial neonatal convulsions
	Myoclonic epilepsy (may be benign or severe)
	Vitamin B6 (pyridoxine) dependency
Infancy	Myoclonic epilepsy (may be benign or severe)
1–12 months	West's syndrome (see p. 32; pp. 105–6)
Early childhood	Febrile seizures (see Chapter 9)
(1–5 years)	Lennox–Gastaut syndrome
Later childhood	Typical absence epilepsy (petit mal epilepsy)
(5–10 years)	Benign partial epilepsy with centro-temporal spikes.
	Benign partial epilepsy with occipital spikes/paroxysms
	Landau–Kleffner syndrome
Adolescence	Juvenile myoclonic epilepsy
	Grand mal seizures on awakening
	Typical absence epilepsy of adolescence

The 'causes' of these syndromes, insofar as they are known, are considered in Chapter 3.

anti-epileptic treatment, and to predict most accurately the outcome. However, it must be understood that even if an epilepsy syndrome is identified, this does not necessarily give any information about the underlying cause of the epilepsy. Indeed, one syndrome such as West's syndrome (p. 32; pp. 105–6) may have several more or less well identified causes.

Many of the different epilepsy syndromes begin in childhood, and are best characterized by onset by age (Table 2.1). However, it is important to think in terms of the two great divisions of primary generalized epilepsy, in which the seizure discharge is generalized from the beginning, and location-related epilepsy, in which the seizure begins in one particular part (location) of the cortex, even if the seizure then becomes a secondary generalized one. A location-related epilepsy usually implies some local structural damage to, or disorder of, nerve cells. One example would be seizures following a head injury. Other examples are given in Chapter 3.

Some syndromes have common features and a predictable outcome. For example, some children develop nocturnal partial seizures often occurring at night, and characterized by large EEG spikes over the central and temporal regions of the brain on one side. Others are rather loose collections of a few common characteristics irregularly linked together.

In the opinion of most experts, only about 40–50 per cent of children with epilepsy can be 'put into' an epilepsy syndrome. When these children cannot be 'put into' or classified into an epilepsy syndrome, then the children's epilepsy must be classified according to the seizure type or types that the child is experiencing, and this used as the best basis for prognostic judgement.

The question of inheritance of epilepsy is considered in Chapter 3, but with the advances in genetic research, the classification of epilepsy syndromes may eventually become replaced by specific epilepsy disorders or diseases classified genetically. However, for the time being, the concept of epilepsy syndromes is of some use.

The relationship between types of seizure and types of epilepsy

Figure 2.3 shows three interlocking circles, the area of which is roughly proportional to the frequency of occurrence of various types of seizure. The central circle incorporates tonic–clonic (grand mal) seizures. The left-hand circle contains partial seizures, many of which become secondarily generalized, as indicated by the considerable overlap between the two circles. Most partial seizures arise from some focal area of structural abnormality within the brain. These seizures can be said to be symptomatic of some underlying problem—so-called *symptomatic epilepsy*.

The right-hand circle indicates typical absences (petit mal seizures). About 30 per cent of children with petit mal also have grand mal seizures, as is indicated by the overlap between right hand and centre circles. Such primary generalized epilepsy is not symptomatic of underlying structural brain disease, and may be said to be constitutional or *idiopathic epilepsy*.

The area of the centre circle that is not overlapped by the left and right hand circles contains those subjects who only have tonic–clonic (grand mal) seizures. Such *cryptogenic epilepsy* (epilepsy of hidden

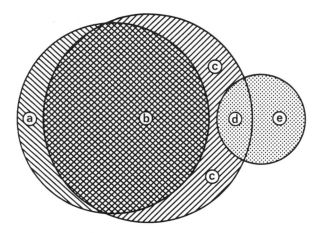

Fig. 2.3 Relation between different types of epileptic seizures and different types of epilepsy. a, partial seizures alone; b, partial seizures evolving to tonic–clonic seizures; c, tonic–clonic seizures of uncertain origin; d, tonic–clonic seizures in association with typical absences; e, typical absences alone. a + b, symptomatic epilepsy; c, cryptogenic epilepsy; d + e, idiopathic epilepsy (primary generalized or constitutional epilepsy).

cause), less common since the advent of sophisticated investigations, should not be called idiopathic. Two possibilities exist—either the petit mal trait was not obvious in childhood, and grand mal seizures are the only manifestation of idiopathic epilepsy, or the seizure discharge from a small lesion becomes generalized so quickly that its initial partial phase is overlooked. It is often difficult to distinguish between the two possibilities even with prolonged EEG recording, unless a seizure actually occurs during the record.

The frequency with which different types of seizure occur

The best information about this comes from studies carried out in general practice. (Table 2.2).

Table 2.2 Classification of types of seizure six months after onset of epilepsy in 564 people (all ages) (data from the National General Practice Study of Epilepsy)

		Per cent
Classifiable		91.0
Unclassifiable		9.0
Generalized seizures		39.0
Tonic–clonic	35.0	
Absences	1.0	
Myoclonic	<1.0	
Other generalized	2.5	
Partial seizures		53.0
Simple	3.0	
Complex	11.0	
Partial evolving to secondarily generalized	27.0	

3 *The causes of epilepsy*

One aspect of human nature is to search for causal links between events. The onset of epileptic seizures in a previously healthy child or adult results in great heart-searching in the family, and raking over past events in an attempt to find some reasons. Yet it has to be admitted that the most careful medical assessment of past events or current state allows a paediatrician or neurologist to assign a cause or causes of epilepsy in only a minority of subjects, and then often on the basis of circumstantial evidence.

Take head injury, for example. If a child is known to have cut her head falling in the playground, and then has her first seizure two weeks later, many parents will link the two events, and attribute the onset of epilepsy to this minor head injury on no basis other than coincidence in time. A minor head injury at work followed some weeks later by a first seizure unfortunately may lead to litigation between employer and employee, as the latter holds that he 'was perfectly all right before the accident'. The association of events in time is, however, no evidence of cause. Severe head injuries may, however, result in the development of epilepsy, so-called post-traumatic epilepsy, as is discussed on pp. 33–5. Somewhere in the continuum of mild to moderate to severe head injuries there must be a zone where there is reasonable doubt as to whether epilepsy was or was not caused by the injury.

The same arguments apply when assessing the effects of a difficult birth and the possible relationship of that to the subsequent development of epilepsy. There is no doubt that a very difficult labour, especially if the baby is small, may cause significant brain damage, severe learning difficulties, cerebral palsy, and epilepsy may result. However, after many difficult or prolonged labours the child develops perfectly normally and twins are no more likely to develop seizures than single births. It used to be thought that forceps or breech deliveries might be blamed for the subsequent development of epilepsy. However, a follow-up study of all children born in one week showed that epilepsy was no more likely to develop after such births than after normal unassisted deliveries. It is now known that in many children born with cerebral palsy or severe learning difficulties there are problems in cerebral development that precede birth. Although sometimes these may be visible on scanning, in other cases the abnormality is no more than a subtle disorder of organization of the developing nerve cells visible only microscopically in tissue obtained at surgical operation or after death. These may, however, be sufficient to cause seizures.

Having given these warnings against uncritically linking life events and the development of epilepsy, what are the factors which can be said, with a fair degree of confidence, to cause epilepsy? The causes are different at different ages. Table 3.1 illustrates this. Some causes, such as a structural congenital brain abnormality may cause seizures in the neonatal period, and the abnormally organized brain may cause seizures throughout life, as is indicated by the long continuing arrow in Table 3.1 Other causes occur only at one age, and their effect then ceases. Metabolic disturbances in the neonatal period, such as hypoglycaemia, are examples of this. Each main group of causes is now explained in detail.

Inheritance

Until about 40 years ago most doctors believed that inheritance was a major factor in causing epilepsy. This belief is still strong amongst the population at large. Doctors are often told 'It can't be epilepsy because there is nothing like that in the family'. These views were held in the past with such force in some states of America and in some Scandinavian countries that it was illegal for people with epilepsy to marry. It is certainly true that genetic factors do play a part in epilepsy, but not an overwhelming part.

There are some genetic diseases in which inheritance is through a *dominant* gene. Genes come in pairs, one from each parent. One member of the pair may always be *dominant* in influencing the structure or biochemistry of the offspring. If a child or adult has the gene, then, in broad terms he or she has the disease, although there are variations in the severity of the disease. One of the parents carrying the gene will therefore not only show the effects of the gene

Table 3.1 Causes of epilepsy at different ages

Cause	Newborn	Infant	Child	Adult
Genetic		‘Idiopathic’ ——————————————→		
		— Lipidoses —————		→
		— Tuberose sclerosis ———		→
			— Neurofibromatosis ———	→
			— Angioma ———————	→
Congenital Anoxia*	At birth ——————			→
		Febrile convulsions ———		→
Trauma	At birth ——————			→
				Stroke ——————→
			Head injury ———————	→
			Intracranial surgery ———	→
				Head injury ——————→
				Intercranial surgery ——→
Tumours			Tumours ———————	Tumours ——————→
Infectious diseases (bacteria, viruses, parasites)	Meningitis ————			
		Meningitis ——————	Meningitis ——————	Meningitis ————→
		Encephalitis ——————	Encephalitis ——————	Encephalitis ————→
			Abscess ——————	Abscess ————————→
				Chronic renal failure —→
Acquired metabolic disease	Hypoglycaemia Hypercalcaemia			
Alcohol				Chronic alcohol abuse —→
Degenerative disorders				Dementia ——————→

*Reduction of oxygen supply to the brain

himself or herself, but will transmit the effective gene to, on average, half his or her children. Tuberous sclerosis and neurofibromatosis, both disorders affecting the structure of nerve cells and surrounding tissue, are transmitted in this way.

There are other genetic diseases in which the gene is *recessive*. In recessive inheritance, the effects of the gene are only expressed if a child has a *double* dose of the relevant gene—one abnormal gene from each parent. The parents, although themselves *carriers*, do not show the abnormality as the other member of their pair of genes is normal. There are certain rare disorders of metabolism of the brain, collectively known as the lipidoses, which are inherited by recessive genes. Fatty substances known as lipids are important constituents of the membranes surrounding the nerve cells. A disorder of the structure and function of the cell membrane may well lead to paroxysmal discharge of nerve cells—an epileptic seizure.

It must be stressed that these diseases are rare. They have been mentioned first only because the mechanism of their inheritance is most clearly understood.

There is, however, also good evidence that primary generalized idiopathic epilepsy, as defined on p. 23, is also inherited. In order to explain this, it is easier to trace back from a child with epilepsy to his parents, rather than first considering the chances of a prospective parent with epilepsy having an epileptic child, a problem which is considered on p. 22. The characteristic EEG is seen in about 40 per cent of brothers and sisters of children with primary generalized epilepsy, even if these brothers and sisters have not had any apparent seizures. That is to say, the abnormality which causes the abnormal EEG record is inherited, but this abnormality is not necessarily *expressed* in clinically apparent seizures. A smaller proportion of the parents of children with primary generalized epilepsy will also show the characteristic EEG changes. We know from following the children with these EEG changes that the characteristic discharges become much less frequent with age, so the absence of discharges in adult life does not mean that the parent did not have unrecorded and unapparent discharges in childhood. From mathematical studies of the proportion of the abnormal EEG records of many families with primary generalized epilepsy, it is possible to calculate that the pattern of inheritance is probably that of a dominant gene.

Energetic research studies are ongoing in several centres to identify the gene. It will probably turn out that there is more than one gene, each giving a similar clinical picture. This has already been shown to be true for the much more clearly defined disorder of tuberouss sclerosis, a disorder in which there are nests of abnormally developed nerve cells and their supporting cells (known as *glial* cells), some of them calcified and some sufficiently large to be seen on a brain scan. It is now known that *two* dominant genes on separate chromosomes can result in what appears to be an identical picture. (A *chromosome* is the microscopically visible structure within the nucleus of a cell which contains the genetic material—the DNA.)

As we have already explained, for a child to show an abnormality in cases of dominant inheritance, only one member of the pair of relevant genes (one from the father and one from the mother) needs to be abnormal. However, the effects of other gene pairs may to some extent succeed in suppressing this gene from expressing itself in obvious seizures. This means that about only one third of the children to whom it is transmitted will have seizures. Furthermore, even if the gene is expressed in seizures, the result may only be a few absence seizures in childhood.

The variability in clinical expression of the genetic abnormality accounts for the occurrence of primary generalized epilepsy in a child of parents neither of whom has ever had a known seizure. In such an instance one assumes that one parent does indeed have the gene, and, had an EEG been recorded in his or her childhood, the typical EEG discharge would have been seen.

Another aspect is the inheritance of a *convulsive threshold*. As explained on pp. 3–4, any one of us can be made to have a seizure if the stimulus is strong enough, and some of us do at lower levels of stimulus—at lower thresholds—than others. The inheritance of this level of threshold is probably *polygenic*—that is to say, several genes, some recessive and some dominant, interact to produce the final result. Another example of polygenic inheritance is height. Tall parents tend to have tall children, but height is not determined by a single gene.

This inherited convulsive threshold is a background, as it were, to the whole of the area in Table 3.1 to the right of the first column. It influences even those cases in which epilepsy clearly seems to be secondary to some obvious cause, such as a severe head injury causing local cortical scarring. Head injuries obviously are not inherited as such. Nevertheless there is a slight tendency for those who develop epilepsy after head injury to have a family history of epilepsy more often than those who do not develop epilepsy after what may be regarded as a comparable injury. What is being inherited here, through a number of different genes, is a lower-than-average convulsive threshold. The children of such head-injured parents are not likely to have seizures unless some additional cerebral damage affects them. It would be an unlikely family in which two members suffered severe head injuries, so that the risk of 'inheriting' epilepsy from a parent with epilepsy secondary to some structural brain damage is small. It follows that one good reason for a paediatrician or neurologist to do his or her best to find a 'cause' for epilepsy is so that they can best advise about the risk of brothers or sisters or daughters or sons being affected.

There is, however, one group of people in whom inherited and acquired characteristics interplay in a complex way. The tendency to febrile convulsions is inherited, through one or more genes, as explained on pp. 142–3.

A febrile convulsion, if very prolonged (lasting longer than 20–30 minutes), may rarely damage one or other temporal lobes of the brain through lack of oxygen occurring during the seizure. The scar in the temporal lobe may then act as a focus from which paroxysmal discharge—seizures—spread in later childhood and adult life.

The first duty of a doctor asked by a young couple, one of whom has epilepsy, about the chances of any child of theirs having epilepsy, is to characterize the seizure type as accurately as possible, using the description of the seizures and the EEG. If it is clear that the prospective parent is having partial seizures, or generalized seizures which have a clear focal onset, either clinically or demonstrated on the EEG then, as explained on p. 22, these seizures are almost certainly secondary to some area of cortical scarring or developmental abnormalities. The risk of any child of this marriage having epilepsy is only moderately higher than the risk of the population at large. It is, however, somewhat higher than the risk of the average child because of the inheritance of the convulsive threshold. If it is clear that the prospective parent has primary generalized epilepsy, then we have to say that about half his or her children will carry the gene, but only about one child in six will have definite seizures. The chances of epilepsy being a *significant* problem in the life of a child of a parent with primary generalized epilepsy is no more than of the order of five per cent, the others perhaps having only a minor EEG abnormality if that is specifically looked for.

This is a complex section of this book, and there is one final complexity. A small fraction of the genetic material (DNA) is carried outside the nucleus in small particles in the cell known as *mitochondria*. These are *only* derived from the maternal ovum, not being present in sperm. There are therefore a few rare disorders in which inheritance is only through the maternal line. Some of these are associated with epilepsy.

Congenital malformation

Some congenital abnormalities (present at birth) are not inherited. For example, the abnormalities in the limbs of the children whose mothers had taken the drug thalidomide during pregnancy are congenital and will not be passed on to their children, as the thalidomide affected the developing cells in the limbs without, (although there continues to be some debate), causing any mutations in the baby's own ovaries or testes. Other congenital abnormalities may have an inherited basis.

One congenital abnormality relevant to epilepsy is a maldevelopment of blood vessels known as an angioma. The abnormal vessels may be either arterial, venous, or capillary. Sometimes a clot or thrombus forms in one or more of the abnormal vessels, exacerbating the situation. One type of capillary angioma of the brain is associated with a similar malformation of blood vessels in the skin of the upper part of the face—the Sturge–Weber syndrome. Children with this particular combination of angiomatous abnormalities have a high probability of developing seizures.

More common than angiomas as a cause of epilepsy are disorders of migration of nerve cells during fetal development, so some end up in the wrong place, the wrong layer of the brain, or with the wrong connections. They are congenital abnormalities, but unlike a harelip, for example, externally invisible. The causes of such disorders are not known, but some probably have a genetic basis. The more obvious are visible on magnetic resonance imaging (p. 74). This sort of abnormal brain development may cause seizures and fits in the first few weeks or months of life, including infantile spasms (West's syndrome).

Anoxia

Anoxia means lack of sufficient oxygen, an essential component of the normal ongoing chemistry of the cell. Cerebral nerve cells are amongst the highest consumers of oxygen in the body, as reflected in the fact that a quarter of all arterial blood goes to the brain. If the oxygen supply is cut off, then damage to nerve cells occurs after a few minutes. Some die, but others are damaged in such a way that they may paroxysmally discharge in subsequent life.

Anoxia may occur at birth. During each uterine contraction in a prolonged labour the fetal heart rate slows, and the supply of oxygenated blood to the brain is reduced. The umbilical cord may become tightly wound around the baby's neck. The placenta may separate prematurely. After birth, for a variety of reasons, the child may not breathe for a few minutes. These are four examples of how anoxic brain damage can occur at birth. If severe, the brain damage results in severe learning difficulties, cerebral palsy, or epilepsy. However, as has already been mentioned, the cause of these three is often due to antenatal factors rather than problems with the birth itself.

Anoxia also occurs in febrile convulsions, as has already been discussed. During a seizure the oxygen requirements of brain nerve cells are enormously increased, and yet the resulting convulsion interferes with normal respiration, so that the blood leaving the lungs picks up insufficient oxygen. The combination of excessive demand and inadequate supply may on rare occasions result in anoxic damage to cerebral nerve cells. The nerve cells which seem most susceptible to damage, at the age at which febrile convulsions occur, are in the temporal lobe.

A stroke is usually due to an obstruction to an arterial vessel to one particular part of the brain, so nerve cells in the territory supplied by the blocked vessel either die as a result of lack of oxygen, or become damaged in such a way that they may form a focus for paroxysmal discharges later. Most strokes occur in late adult life, and cerebrovascular disease accounts for much of the epilepsy beginning in old age. Occasionally, however, a stroke may occur in a young adult or even in a child.

Trauma

Damage to cerebral nerve cells may occur through physical trauma. In war time, head injuries due to penetrating injuries from shrapnel are a potent source of epilepsy. About 45 per cent of survivors develop later seizures. In civilian life most head injuries are closed—that is to say there is no penetration of the skull. However, the impact of the head with the dashboard or road in road traffic injuries may cause the later development of post-traumatic epilepsy.

Professor Bryan Jennett of Glasgow has done a great deal to sort out the factors in a head injury that are most likely to cause later epilepsy (Fig. 3.1). The first is the duration of the post-traumatic amnesia. This is the name given to the period after a head injury when patients, although conscious, are not recording in their memory on-going events, even though they may seem to be behaving rationally at the time. A typical story is for a man to have no recollection of relatives visiting him in hospital, even though he talked and joked with them. The duration of post-traumatic amnesia may vary from a few minutes, when the term 'concussion' is often loosely applied, to many weeks or even months. The mechanism of the amnesia is not known, but a useful analogy is to consider a blancmange in a mould (the brain in the skull). A vigorous tap or shaking of the mould may cause oscillations so violent within the blancmange that cracks appear within its structure, even though the mould remains intact. Such shearing forces can be demonstrated within the brains of animals subject to experimental head injuries. The longer the duration of

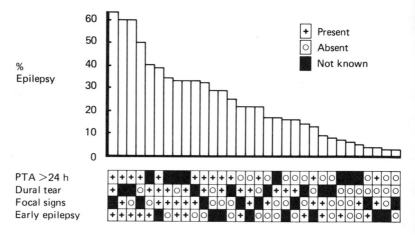

Fig. 3.1 Incidence of late epilepsy after compound depressed fracture of the skull in which three or four factors were known. (Redrawn from W.B. Jennett (1975). *Epilepsy after non-missile head injuries.* Heinemann, London, with kind permission.)

post-traumatic amnesia, the greater the chance of the development of later epilepsy.

The second factor which Professor Jennett found to be important was the presence of focal neurological signs, such as changes in the reflexes, after the injury. Presumably these just reflect a greater degree of disruption of the brain.

The third factor was the presence of local damage to the cortical surface of the brain, as judged by the presence of a tear in the dura—the membrane covering the brain. The impact of the head on a sharp corner may cause a depressed fracture, with fragments of bone tearing the dura and becoming embedded in the cortex.

Professor Jennett found that if all three factors were present in one case (a prolonged amnesia of more than 24 hours after the head injury, focal neurological signs, and a dural tear), then there was a 40 per cent chance of developing epileptic seizures later. If none of these factors was present the risk was about two per cent.

Professor Jennett also noted that some head-injured patients had a seizure in the first week after the injury. The occurrence of such an event—perhaps the marker of an inherited low convulsive threshold or of extensive cortical damage—was a potent predictor of late post-traumatic epilepsy. A seizure in the first week, accompanied by a long post-traumatic amnesia and focal neurological signs was followed by later seizures in 60 per cent of cases, even if the dura were not torn.

There are other types of brain injury apart from those caused by the ubiquitous road traffic and industrial accidents. Cerebral trauma also occurs, unavoidably, during cranial operations. For example, small balloon-like swellings called 'aneurysms' on arteries at the base of the brain are never, by themselves, responsible for epilepsy. In order to avoid the risk of haemorrhage, operation may be advised. The surgeon, in approaching the aneurysms in order to clip the neck of the 'balloons', has to handle and retract, albeit very gently, normal brain. Unfortunately seizures may follow such handling of cerebral tissues.

Tumours

A tumour arising within the brain understandably causes great anxiety–perhaps more so than with tumours elsewhere in the body, as a brain tumour may appear to strike at the very centre of one's soul and being. Many people with simple headaches due to anxiety or stress believe that they have a brain tumour which is causing their headache. However, the incidence of primary tumour (see below) is very low (10 per 100 000 per year). It is, however, true that tumours can cause epilepsy. This is much more likely to happen in adults than in children.

Brain tumours are either primary or secondary. A secondary tumour is one that has been carried in the blood to the brain from another site. Cancers of the lung (bronchus) or breast are by far the most common of these. Usually the site of the original cancer is known, and the appearance of seizures in such a patient is an ominous sign indicating that a secondary tumour has arisen within the brain. Sometimes, however, the original cancer has not been discovered at the time of the first seizure, and a careful clinical examination will reveal a small tell-tale lump in the breast, or the lung cancer will be seen on a chest X-ray.

Primary tumours of the brain do not arise in nerve cells. They either arise in the supporting cells between nerve cells which play an active role in their nutrition (glial cells) or in the meninges, the covering membranes of the brain. These tumours are called gliomas and meningiomas. There are other types of primary cerebral tumours, such as those arising from the cells lining the cavities of the brain, or from blood vessels, but these are rare.

Primary brain tumours are not like cancer of the breast, or bowel, or bronchus. They show no tendency to develop blood-borne secondary deposits in other organs. This is fortunate, but there are other characteristics which hinder effective treatment. The gliomas infiltrate normal brain extensively, so there is no apparent margin beyond which one can be quite certain that no abnormal cells have reached. This makes recurrence after surgical excision very likely. Meningiomas, however, are encapsulated tumours, and can often be removed completely, with a good chance of complete eradication. However, meningiomas often have an extensive blood supply, so complete removal may be technically very difficult.

Infectious diseases

Bacterial meningitis can damage the brain at any age from the newborn period to old age. Vigorous and early treatment with antibiotics and corticosteroid drugs nearly always prevents damage to the cortex, which lies immediately under the meningeal covering of the brain. However, if the treatment is delayed, or the organism is resistant to the antibiotic chosen, the damaged cortical cells may act as seizure foci in subsequent years. Meningitis due to tuberculosis is particularly likely to result in later epilepsy.

A bacterial brain abscess usually now results from blood-borne bacteria which are deposited in the cerebral hemispheres in a patient who is acutely ill with septicaemia. However, most blood-borne bacteria from an infection are filtered out from venous blood as this passes through the capillaries of the lungs. An exception occurs if there is a hole between right and left sides of the heart. Some bacteria may then pass directly from the venous circulation into the left ventricle and into the cerebral circulation. This accounts for the high incidence of cerebral abscess in those with these types of congenital heart disease.

An abscess may also form by direct extension into the brain from a local infection—for example, severe middle ear suppuration or frontal sinusitis may cause abscesses respectively in the temporal or frontal lobes of the brain.

Acute abscesses can certainly cause epileptic seizures, but, even if successfully treated by drainage and by antibiotics, further seizures may arise from the scar. In an attempt to avoid this, many surgeons now excise totally the capsule of the abscess rather than simply aspirate the pus.

Viral meningitis is a self-limiting illness, and epilepsy does not occur after this. Sometimes, however, the viruses are present within the substance of the brain, rather than remaining confined to the surface. This is called encephalitis, and seizures may result. Two of the more common viruses causing seizures in this way are the herpes and cytomegaloviruses. Cytomegalovirus usually affects the fetal (unborn baby's) brain, and the herpes virus usually affects infants, young children, and adults. The HIV virus can also cause seizures, either by itself or, through depressing the immune system, allowing invasion of the brain by other viruses, and often by a small organism known as *Toxoplasma*.

Some viruses behave in a very strange way in the brain. Measles, for example, is an illness which affects nearly all children without significant late effects. The illness is terminated by the production of antibodies. A tiny number of children, however, do not succeed in eradicating the virus from their brains, and, some years later a new measles-related illness begins—sub-acute sclerosing pan-encephalitis—in which seizures and mental deterioration are prominent. Fortunately this is now becoming very rare with the wider use of measles vaccine.

Parasites can also cause epilepsy. The pork tapeworm *Taenia solium* may cause epilepsy if the cystic stage of the tapeworm, usually found in pigs, occurs in the muscles and brain of man. In developing countries, calcified cysts are found in the brains of many of the rural population and this disorder, cysticercosis, and tuberculosis accounts for a lot of the greater incidence of epilepsy in such populations. The dog tapeworm *Toxocara* has also been incriminated in the development of epilepsy, though with less certain evidence. Toxoplasmosis, possibly acquired through infection *in utero* from domestic animals is certainly associated with seizures.

Creutzfeldt–Jakob disease is a rare disorder caused by an infectious agent which is not a bacteria or a virus. One route of transmission is through surgical instruments (ordinary sterilization does not kill it) or through tissue transplantation (for example, corneal transplantation). It is related to 'mad-cow' disease (BSE, bovine spongiform encephalopathy). Affected adults may have seizures as part of the serious neurological illness.

Acquired metabolic disorders

The pathways of chemical metabolism in the newborn are very unstable and vast changes in the serum concentrations of various substances can occur. A blood glucose concentration sufficiently low (hypoglycaemia) to cause seizures, for example, cannot be induced in older children or adults by starvation, or indeed by any means other than the injection of insulin. However, severe hypoglycaemia resulting in seizures may be seen in the newborn, particularly in premature infants, or in babies born to diabetic mothers.

Seizures due to a low serum calcium are also fairly frequent in the newborn period. One cause is early feeding with cow's milk, which is very rich in phosphates, and which results in increased renal excretion of calcium and subsequent low levels of calcium in the blood.

In later stages of life, other acquired metabolic disorders may cause seizures. Chronic renal failure used to be one of the more common causes, but dialysis and successful transplantation of kidneys has reduced the frequency of seizures due to this cause.

Alcohol

Alcohol may undoubtedly precipitate seizures in those who already have had previous seizures. This aspect is discussed on p. 42.

There is also an association between chronic alcohol abuse and the occurrence of fits even when sober. Those who drink alcohol to excess are usually aware that they are running the risk of cirrhosis of the liver, but not many realize that chronic alcoholism can result in loss of cerebral nerve cells, seizures, and impairment of intellect.

Degenerative disorders

As advances in knowledge occur, fewer and fewer diseases will be assigned to this non-specific group. Creutzfeld–Jakob disease, the human equivalent of 'mad cow' disease for example, used to be regarded as degenerative , before it was shown to be caused by an infective agent. Pre-senile dementia (Alzheimer's disease), in which the cerebral nerve cells gradually become fewer in number, is associated with seizures. Some cases are inherited, and almost certainly in most there is a biochemical abnormality responsible for this loss of nerve cells, and, hopefully, when this has been identified, some sort of pharmacological treatment will be possible. This sequence of events has already occurred in Parkinson's disease. This was regarded as a degenerative disorder until 30 years ago. A defect in the metabolism of a transmitter called dopamine was identified, and a suitable drug (L-dopa) produced. A number of degenerative disorders which start in childhood (including one called Batten's disease) present with frequent seizures.

How common are the individual causes of epilepsy?

Table 3.2 shows the causes of epilepsy that could be defined, with a fair degree of confidence, in each of two studies. The way in which the subjects were selected was different in each study, but the final figure—the proportion in which a cause for epilepsy could be defined—varied within narrow limits, between only 34.5 per cent and 39.0 per cent.

The fact that 61.0–65.5 per cent of people with epilepsy have no discernible cause for their seizures certainly does not mean that the remainder have 'idiopathic' epilepsy as defined on p. 22. Since

Table 3.2 Causes of epilepsy in two community studies (per cent)

	USA	UK
Perinatal/congenital	8.0	–
Trauma	5.5	3.0
Vascular	10.9	15.0
Tumours	4.1	6.0
Infection	2.5	2.0
Degenerative	3.5	6.0
Alcohol	(excluded)	7.0
Uncertain (cryptogenic plus idiopathic)	65.5	61.0

USA Data from Olmstead County study (1993)
UK Data from National General Practitioner Study of Epilepsy (1990)
The most common degenerative disorders is Alzheimer's disease

the advent of magnetic resonance imaging we know that a large proportion of subjects with such 'cryptogenic' epilepsy (epilepsy of hidden cause), have minor structural changes in the brain—very commonly zones of atrophy in one or other temporal lobe. Because of the expense and relative novelty of the procedure, many of the subjects about whom information appears in Table 3.2 never had such an imaging study. More recent studies show that nearly 90 per cent of those with temporal lobe epilepsy, for example, will have abnormalities on magnetic resonance imaging, though these abnormalities may be very minor, and only detectable with careful measurements on the scan.

Precipitants of seizures

Whatever the 'cause', most people with epilepsy analyse their day to day lives in an attempt to detect factors which precipitate seizures.

Virtually every conceivable life event may be blamed by some people with epilepsy, who may become overly obsessional about avoiding factors they consider important. For example, a man had each of his two seizures on railway trains. He firmly believes that in some way trains make him have seizures. It is likely that this occurrence is just coincidental, but we cannot be entirely sure that he is wrong!

There are, however, a number of factors which do seem to precipitate seizures in at least some people with epilepsy.

Sleep and lack of sleep

The electroencephalogram (EEG) is discussed fully on pp. 61–72. At this stage, it is only necessary to know that it records the changes in voltage resulting from activity of cerebral nerve cells. The EEGs of people without epilepsy change during the passage from normal wakefulness, through drowsiness, to sleep. Sleep is not constant, as judged by body movements and EEG patterns, throughout the night. At various intervals one pattern of brain waves occur in association with rapid movements of the eyes. Through waking patients at this time we know that it is during this stage of sleep that dreams occur.

The changing electrical activity of the brain during drowsiness and sleep may allow seizure discharges to 'escape'. Indeed, those analysing EEGs hope that their patients drop off to sleep during the procedure as the possibility of recording an abnormality is considerably enhanced.

Some subjects have all or virtually all the seizures whilst asleep—but they can never be entirely sure that a daytime attack will not occur. A follow-up study of one group of people with 'nocturnal' epilepsy showed that about a third had a daytime seizure in the next five years. The effects of depriving people of sleep have also been studied by keeping volunteers continuously awake, or by waking them up every time the EEG showed the pattern of rapid eye movement sleep. In each case EEGs on subsequent undisturbed nights showed that the subjects were catching up on the rapid eye movement sleep they had missed. Deprivation of sleep, therefore, has been shown to alter cerebral electrical activity, and it is not surprising that this is another factor in precipitating seizures. In practical terms, repeatedly staying up late may precipitate seizures in young adults.

Alcohol

One of the most common reasons for staying up later than usual is to go to a party, where alcohol may be drunk. The social use of alcohol depends largely on its ability to remove inhibiting factors in our personalities and conversation, thereby making us perhaps more interesting and amusing. A similar removal of inhibition of an epileptic focus may allow a seizure to occur. Often, however, the seizure occurs during the 'hangover', at a time when the blood alcohol is falling, or near zero. It is probable that other changes in body chemistry, particularly in the distribution of water within and outside cells, plays a part in causing such seizures. Over-hydration of experimental animals with epilepsy may precipitate seizures, so there are grounds for believing that large quantities of beer, containing both alcohol and much water, may be more likely to precipitate an attack than moderate use of wine or spirits.

Menstruation

Some women gain three or four pounds (1–2 kg) in weight in the few days preceding their menstrual period. This gain is largely fluid, manifested by feeling bloated, with distended, sore breasts. Some women with epilepsy, particularly those with partial seizures, may notice an increase in frequency of seizures at the same time. It is not known if water retention is the responsible factor, or whether there is some more complicated hormonal cause. Dehydration with diuretic drugs has been used in attempts to abolish clusters of seizures occurring in relation to menstruation, but with limited success.

The weight gain associated with oral contraception does not seem to precipitate seizures. Oral contraception for women with epilepsy is satisfactory, provided that they understand the interactions between the pill and anti-epileptic drugs explained on p. 95.

Stress and worry

It is impossible to quantify stress and worry. Problems perceived as molehills by some may be mountains to others. A period of hard work at school or office, or a time of emotional unhappiness at home, is often associated with an increased number of seizures. A vicious circle may arise, whereby stress and worry precipitate seizures, which in themselves cause further anxiety and hence further seizures. Sometimes an increased number of seizures leads to some crisis in employment, and the anxiety this causes results in a further deterioration in both epilepsy and job prospects.

Mood

Mothers of young children with epilepsy can sometimes tell from their child's mood and behaviour that they are 'building up to a fit'. Adults with epilepsy may experience a peculiar feeling of heaviness or depression on the morning of the days of their seizures. Occasionally elation rather than depression is reported. It is impossible to decide whether these emotional changes cause the seizures, whether both the mood and the seizures are caused by some common factor, or whether the change in mood is in some way produced by a limited paroxysmal discharge that finally erupts into an obvious seizure.

Other illnesses

Any one with epilepsy may have a seizure in relation to a severe other illness such as pneumonia. In children with epilepsy, fever may precipitate seizures, but it is important to retain the distinction between these and febrile convulsions (Chapter 9).

Drugs

Some chemical compounds are so powerful that they will cause seizures in most of those exposed. On p. 3 we gave the example of the war gas which has actually been used in some units to induce seizures in those with severe depression as an alternative to electroconvulsive therapy. In this case the seizure is the required effect, but in all other instances seizures complicating drug therapy are very much an unwanted effect.

Antidepressant drugs of the tricyclic group, including amitryptiline (for example, Tryptizol, Saroten, Domical) and nortryptyline (for example, Allegron, Aventyl) are amongst those which clearly lower the convulsive threshold and precipitate seizures. Other offenders include phenothiazines, isoniazid, and high doses of penicillin. Excessive doses of insulin precipitate seizures through hypoglycaemia (low blood sugar). Any of these drugs may precipitate a first seizure or exacerbate established epilepsy.

Other drugs may precipitate seizures in those with epilepsy on anti-epileptic medication by interfering with the metabolism of these drugs.

Finally, it should be remembered that *withdrawal* of some drugs, particularly barbiturates, may precipitate seizures.

Other precipitants—reflex epilepsy

More specific than any of the precipitants so far discussed are the stimuli which result in so-called reflex epilepsy. Some young people have seizures induced by flashing lights, as in a discotheque, and this can be studied on an EEG. In most of us, an obvious wave can be recorded from the back of the head (the occipital region) if a light is flashed in the eyes. With repeated flashes, these waves follow the flash frequency. At a critical frequency in a young person with photosensitive epilepsy, a totally different response of multiple spikes and waves—the *photoconvulsive response*—occurs, and a seizure may be induced. This of course is a laboratory situation, but seizures may result, in photosensitive children, from flickering light reflected from water, or by the interruption of steady light filtered through trees observed from a moving car.

The most common type of photosensitivity now encountered is *television epilepsy*. Experiments have shown that it is the normal sweep of the spots that make up the picture from side to side and down the face of the tube that is responsible, and not any malfunction of vertical picture or horizontal line hold. Susceptible children are most at risk when the screen occupies a considerable proportion of the visual field, as will occur if the size of the screen is large, and the child sits close to it, or approaches it to change the programme. The chances of seizures occurring are lessened by sitting far away from the screen. It may also help to reduce contrast between the screen and surroundings by placing the set near a lamp.

It has also been shown that the photoconvulsive response cannot be elicited if only one eye is exposed to the flashing light. It makes sense, therefore, for susceptible children to cover one eye if they approach the set. Remote programme selection by infra-red control is useful for such children. Both colour and monochrome television sets induce seizures, which are invariably generalized, though they may sometimes be of very short duration—just a few myoclonic jerks of arms and trunk muscles. Video games may also precipitate seizures. However, although text on computer screens is occasionally associated with seizures, the problem is far less, and only occasional seizures have been reported.

Another type of visual reflex epilepsy occurs on looking at patterns such as squares of linoleum tiling. This may be regarded as typical of the highly specific reflex epilepsies occurring in a very few patients in which seizures may be induced by, for example, reading, hearing music (sometimes by only one particular phrase), or by performing mental arithmetic. The perception of such external stimuli must result in a particular pattern of nerve cell activity—this is presumably in part how we recognize tunes and words. One can only imagine that this particular set of activity in susceptible people acts as a specific template which, like a key in a lock, unlooses a seizure.

Non-specific stimuli—such as a loud noise, or a startle, however caused, may induce myoclonic jerks, and occasionally a generalized tonic–clonic seizure. This type of epilepsy is seen as an inherited feature in some strains of mice, and provides a model for the investigation of the physiology of such seizures, and a model for trying out the potential effectiveness of new anti-epileptic drugs.

4 *The first seizure and the diagnosis of epilepsy*

Anyone reading this book who has been present at the first grand mal seizure of a child or other relative will remember the sense of shock and feeling of incompetence at coping with a totally unforeseen situation. A common story is for parents to be woken by the stertorous breathing or grunting of a child in the next bedroom. They go to him, thinking usually that he is having a bad dream, and find him staring, unresponsive, convulsing, and perhaps blue. Few if any parents can cope calmly with such a scene. It is usual for the family doctor to be telephoned at once, and, if there is any delay in his arrival, for an ambulance to be summoned as well. Many parents subsequently confess that they thought their child was dying, so they are acting in an entirely rational way. Almost invariably, however, by the time the family doctor or ambulance has arrived, the seizure is over, the child is sleeping peacefully, and the adults are making tea. But they will not sleep again that night. Many—though not all—are immediately aware of the nature of what they have just seen, and all the worries which this book is attempting to put into perspective crowd their minds.

Although the first seizure can occur anywhere and at any time, another common scenario is for the first seizure to occur in a young woman in the company of her friends or at work. In this case, the lack of ready access to the family doctor, whose name and telephone number is unlikely to be known to the bystanders, results in an ambulance being almost invariably called, and the unfortunate young woman being rushed off to hospital. She will recover consciousness either in the ambulance or in the Accident and Emergency Department of the hospital. To the confusion invariably consequent to the generalized seizure must be added the feeling of 'What on earth has happened to me, and how have I finished up here on a stretcher with strangers peering at me?' Obviously, therefore, although ambulance services are rather prickly on this point, a friend should accompany her to hospital—not only to provide moral support when recovery of consciousness occurs but also to give an accurate account of events to the hospital staff. In this case, the diagnosis of a tonic–clonic seizure is clear, but in others matters are not so straightforward. It is important to distinguish between an epileptic seizure and some other event which may initially seem to be one. Patients may speak in terms of a 'black-out', 'funny turn', or 'blank spell', and we have to do our best to analyse the cause.

What will the family doctor or Accident and Emergency doctor do?

Apart from listening carefully to the story given by the person and any eyewitness, what else will the doctor do?

She will examine her patient not only to make sure that everything is generally well–for example, that breathing is unobstructed—but she will also ascertain if there are any focal (localized) neurological signs, which may give her a clue to the cause of the seizure. Though she is not likely to find anything abnormal at this stage, there may be some minor signs such as an asymmetry of the reflexes. She will then question the relatives or other witnesses, and satisfy herself that what has just occurred was indeed a seizure, and not some other event of the type discussed later in this chapter. Rarely, the first seizure is an early manifestation of an acute and important illness such as meningitis or encephalitis. If she suspects that this might be the case, she will of course arrange immediate admission to hospital. More often, all that is necessary is for her to give a tablet or injection of diazepam (Valium), which is sufficient to raise the seizure threshold (see p. 29) and make a second seizure less likely for some hours. This will give everyone time to collect their thoughts and decide on the long-term policy decisions, including the possible needs for referral to a specialist, for investigation, and for institution of anti-epileptic treatment.

Is referral to a specialist necessary?

Most referrals occur not because family doctors are uncertain as to whether a patient has had a seizure or not, nor because they are seriously concerned in every case about the possibility of serious underlying disease, but for the following reasons:

- People do not like being told they have had an epileptic seizure. One survey showed that this difficult task is left to the hospital doctor in about half the cases.

- People with epilepsy themselves very often feel that some sort of special test is necessary to 'prove' the diagnosis. This point is discussed in relation to the EEG on p. 7. It must be very difficult to accept the diagnosis, with all its social implications, when it is made on the basis of a 30-second description given to a doctor by a relative or bystander. Somehow it does not seem 'scientific' enough, and yet paediatricians and neurologists place enormous weight on the recounted stories.

- People with epilepsy are very concerned to discover the 'cause' of their epilepsy. As Table 3.2 shows, a cause is often not found, but most people think in terms of a single cause, which they believe, if eradicated, will result in the problem being solved once and for all. Occasionally, of course, an important treatable cause *is* found, and usually special tests are indeed necessary to show this. The difficulty lies in deciding which patients should be so investigated.

- Traditional medical textbooks accentuate the unusual and 'interesting' causes of epilepsy, at the expense of the more usual patients. Family doctors, educated partly by these books, tend to play safe and refer if referral centres are available.

- The necessary decisions are quite complex. There are three possible preliminary diagnoses—seizure, not seizure, and may be seizure; two policies about investigation—to be arranged or not; and four possible outcomes—treatment, no treatment, adoption of a wait-and-see policy, and referral to another specialist. We do have some sympathy with our colleagues in primary care, when all these combinations are considered, and can readily understand why so many patients are referred.

What will the paediatrician or neurologist do?

The analysis of 'funny turns' or 'blackouts' of one sort or another makes up a considerable proportion of the work of a neurologist and quite a bit of the work of a paediatrician. Their first concern is to obtain as accurate as possible an account of the events which led up to and occurred at the time of a seizure. People who have lost consciousness cannot themselves say what happened while they were unconscious. However, people will be able to give important information about what they were doing and how they felt before loss of consciousness, and how they felt when they first recovered, but the neurologist will want to know what was happening during the time that consciousness was disturbed. For this reason an eye-witness account is essential. Information must be asked about:

- What time of day was it?

- What was the person doing before the attack?

- What were the events leading up to the seizure(s)?

- Did the seizure or attack occur without warning, or were there initial symptoms suggestive of an aura (p. 19) or of a simple faint (syncope) (p. 50)?

- What precisely did the child or person look like or do during the seizure?

- How long did the seizure or attack last?

- What did the person look like and do afterwards?

If the patient or eye-witness is unable to recall accurately exactly what happened during the seizure, then it is useful to ask the eye-witness to show the doctor what sort of 'jerking' or shaking occurred, but sometimes people are too shy or embarrassed to do this. If repeated attacks occur, and there remains diagnostic difficulty, the potential eye-witness should be given a list of these check points, and encouraged to use a video-camera or cam-corder to record the seizure or attack. This is becoming increasingly useful in the diagnosis of epilepsy, particularly in infants and young children.

It should be possible to make a definite diagnosis of epilepsy or of some other condition on the basis of all this clinical information.

The diagnosis of epilepsy must not be made lightly and if there is doubt then epilepsy should *not* be diagnosed and the doctor should wait for more convincing evidence from further 'attacks' or episodes before making a firm diagnosis. The risk of someone with epilepsy coming to harm from a delay in the diagnosis is small, whereas a diagnosis of epilepsy incorrectly made is nearly always damaging. This damage may be reflected in unfair prejudice and resulting social burden, in addition to the prescription of unnecessary and potentially hazardous medication.

A large number of conditions may be misdiagnosed as epilepsy particularly in children. These are discussed below.

Simple faints (syncope; vasovagal attacks)

The medical name for these is syncope. Many of us have experienced one or more syncopal attacks, very often at school. In syncope, consciousness is disturbed or lost, not because of a paroxysmal discharge of cerebral nerve cells, but because the cerebral nerve cells are silenced by inadequate supply of oxygen through arterial blood.

When a man stands up, his brain is about 15 inches (38 cm) higher than his heart; when he lies down, the two organs are at the same level. When he stands up, therefore, the arterial pressure has to increase so that blood flow to the brain remains unchanged. Normally, this is accompained smoothly by a combination of increased heart rate and by constriction of the blood vessels in the abdomen and legs. Experience informs us of examples of a breakdown in this mechanism. The most familiar is the extreme slowing of the heart-rate produced in some sensitive people by the sight of blood or in response to pain. This cardiac slowing is mediated through the vagal nerve, and the name vasovagal attack is often given to such an episode.

The contraction of leg and thigh muscles during walking normally

Table 4.1 The differences between syncope and seizures

	Syncope	Seizures
Posture	Upright	Any posture
Pallor and sweating	Invariable	Uncommon
Onset	Gradual	Usually sudden
Injury	Rare	Not uncommon
Convulsive jerks	Not uncommon	Common
Incontinence	Unusual	Common
Unconsciousness	Seconds	Minutes
Recovery	Rapid	Often slow
Post-ictal sleep	Rare	Common
Post-ictal confusion	Rare	Common
Precipitating factors	Crowded places	Rare
	Lack of food	
	Sudden pain or fright	

drives venous blood back to the heart. If venous return is insufficient because of immobility—for example, a soldier at attention on parade, or a young girl in assembly at school—then syncope may occur. Such syncope seems to be socially infectious—once a girl or soldier has slumped, others may follow in the next few minutes.

Normally blood returns to the heart from the legs smoothly through the chest and abdomen. During prolonged coughing, or straining while trying to pass a stool, the pressure within the chest is greatly increased, preventing venous return to the heart. What the heart is not getting back, it cannot put out, so this sequence of events again may result in impaired blood-flow to the brain, and syncope.

If the blood vessels in trunk and legs are pleasantly dilated in a hot bath or nice warm bed, suddenly getting up—for example, to answer the telephone—may cause syncope. This may also happen in older people, when they get out of bed at night to pass urine. The situation is more complex in this case because we know that, at the onset of urination, there is a reflex dilatation of blood vessels in the legs. This so-called 'micturition syncope' affects men more than women, not only because they more often have to pass urine at night (because of prostatic enlargement) but because they pass urine standing up.

Syncope may occur in association with certain diseases. For example, in diabetes the nerve fibres controlling the heart rate and the diameter of blood vessels may be diseased, and the normal adjustments to blood pressure to posture may fail to occur. There are other rare diseases of the brain in which a similar failure to control blood pressure occurs. One, which bears some similarity to Parkinson's disease, is known as the Shy–Drager syndrome after the two American neurologists who first described it.

A much more common cause of syncope, however, is medication. Many people take tablets to control high blood pressure. One effect of some of these drugs is to cause syncope on standing up. Some antidepressants, such as imipramine (Tofranil), do the same.

How does the neurologist or paediatrician decide that his patient's blackouts are due to syncope rather than epilepsy? Again, all depends upon the story. The first clue is the circumstances in which the blackout occurred. If it happened at the scene of a road accident, or during a horror movie, syncope is very likely. A common story is for a man to faint while attending his wife's delivery. Syncope virtually never occurs lying down, so if loss of consciousness happens then, a seizure is more likely. Very occasionally, vagal slowing of the heart can be so profound that syncope *does* happen lying down. For example, one of our patients was a woman who was so terrified of dental treatment that she lost consciousness due to syncope even if the dentist started treating her with the chair tilted back almost to the horizontal position.

The next point is the occurrence of pre-syncopal symptoms. Blood flow to the brain is reduced in syncope often for many seconds before consciousness is lost. During that time, the nervous system makes desperate attempts to constrict other blood vessels in order to elevate the central pressure. The constriction of blood vessels in the skin results in pallor, and the associated discharge of the vegetative (non-voluntary) nervous system causes nausea and sweating. The person therefore feels and looks cold, pale, and clammy.

Other points which help distinguish syncope from seizures include limpness, rather than rigidity and/or convulsions during the period of unconsciousness, and usually no incontinence during the event. Recovery of full consciousnesss and orientation is much more rapid after syncope than after a seizure, following which there is usually a period of confusion. Recovery after syncope often rapidly follows assumption of the horizontal position, whether the person falls, or is placed like this, so that the head is on the same level as the heart. This is nature's safety mechanism whereby cerebral blood flow is restored. Occasionally the safety mechanism cannot operate—the position of a hand-basin or lavatory may prevent the limp body falling to the floor. Sometimes the sufferer is supported in a vertical position by well-meaning but ill-advised friends or bystanders. In these cases, cerebral blood flow may fall to such extremely low levels that incontinence, twitching, or a full-blown seizure may occur. This should be regarded as an 'anoxic seizure' rather than a seizure caused by epilepsy.

As an example of the difficulties that this unusual sequence of events can cause, one of us was asked to see a young nurse. Three days after a straightforward appendicectomy, she got up for the first time to go to the ward lavatory. She felt faint as she walked there, and therefore left the door ajar. She felt fainter still as she was sitting on the seat, straining to open her bowels. Before losing consciousness she called another nurse for help. This girl seeing her colleague about to tumble off the seat, held her up to prevent injury. The resulting cerebral anoxia caused an anoxic seizure. An incorrect diagnosis of epilepsy had been made, and her continued employment as a nurse was under threat.

Syncope in adolescents—usually girls—can be very troublesome, and occasionally injury occurs. Physique and life-style seem irrelevant, so the usual advice to take plenty of fresh air and exercise is probably useless. Much more important is to tell the young person to lie down *at once* if she feels the onset of typical pre-syncopal symptoms. Fortunately recurrent episodes are rarely troublesome for more than a year.

Reflex anoxic seizures

These are a type of syncope, but deserve a particular mention as the attacks are frequently misdiagnosed as epileptic seizures. Reflex anoxic seizures (also called pallid syncopal attacks) usually affect young children between 12 months and 4 years of age, but can affect older children and even adults. The attacks are *always* provoked by either a sudden fright, or unexpected pain. This unpleasant experience then stimulates a nerve (the vagus nerve) which causes the heart to slow down or even stop for a few seconds. As a result of this the child becomes pale, then limp, and may even have a brief clonic convulsion. Almost immediately the child will recover, may cry, and then appear sleepy. Within a few minutes the child is usually back to normal. These attacks do not damage the brain or heart, do not need treatment, and usually stop by the age of 5–10 years.

Breath-holding attacks

These attacks occur only in young children, aged usually between one and three years. The typical story is of a child who is frustrated, told off, or spanked. The child becomes angry or upset and will hold their breath. After a few seconds the child becomes blue (cyanosed) because of a lack of oxygen in the blood and loses consciousness, and becomes limp. Because of the reduced oxygen supply to the brain (as the child is not breathing) the child may have some clonic (jerking) movements and wet themselves. The child always starts breathing again and is back to normal within a few minutes. These breath-holding attacks usually stop by the age of 4–5 years.

Other causes of impaired oxygen supply to the brain

Disturbances of cardiac rhythm (cardiac dysrhythmia)

Disturbance of consciousness in syncope is due to failure of blood supply to the brain, due in part to a fall in cardiac output. Cardiac output may also be less than normal if the rhythm of the heart is abnormal. Both very slow and very fast heart rates diminish cardiac output.

The distinction of a disturbance of consciousness due to an abnormality of cardiac rhythm from a seizure is not easy. Occasionally, though, a bystander will note that someone is pulseless or has a very irregular pulse during the attack, and sometimes the sufferer himself notices palpitations before disturbance of consciousness. Cardiac rhythm is easily monitored by electrocardiography. The changes in voltage associated with contraction of the different chambers of the heart are of sufficient amplitude that they can easily be recorded on a cassette recorder for periods of 24 hours, and their occurrence in relation to symptoms analysed. A cardiac cause for disturbance of consciousness has been found in up to one quarter of cases first presenting to neurological clinics with blackouts.

Localized reduction in cerebral blood flow

The changes in blood flow that we have considered so far affect all parts of the brain equally. In older people, arteriosclerotic changes take place in the arteries in the neck and head. There may be a temporary blockage of an artery to one part of the brain by a fragment of chalky deposit or thrombus swept downstream from a larger artery by the flow of blood. Neurologists call these blockages 'transient ischaemic attacks'. In some of these short episodes, muscle weakness or tingling in one or other limb may slightly resemble partial motor or sensory seizures (pp. 14–15). However, although focal motor seizures may arise in the scarred brain in the territory of a permanently blocked artery after a stroke, *transient* ischaemic attacks are associated with transient paralysis rather than convulsions.

In younger people, localized (focal) neurological phenomena occur in *migraine*. In the first stage of a classical migraine attack, arterial spasm occurs, reducing cerebral blood flow focally. It is unclear whether this is primary or secondary to some depression of nerve cell activity. The occipital area is the region most often affected. This results in a hallucination of distorted vision or flashing lights, rather than the formed visual hallucination which may be part of a partial seizure arising in a temporal lobe (p. 16). Occassionally spasm affects the motor or sensory areas of the brain, producing short-lived paralysis or disturbance of sensation, without convulsions, on the opposite side of the body.

Narcolepsy

Any one of us may feel drowsy in a stuffy lecture theatre, or as a passenger on a long car journey. Those suffering from narcolepsy, however, feel an uncontrollable desire to sleep at other times, and may indeed drop off in socially embarrassing circumstances. This unusual symptom may be associated with 'cataplexy'—a sudden loss of postural tone causing collapse without loss of consciousness, often precipitated by strong emotions such as anger or amusement. In a way, these phenomena are nearest to epilepsy, as they presumably result from some paroxysmal disorder of cerebral nerve cells. However, such patients have epileptic seizures no more often than the general population, the EEG whilst awake is always normal, and drugs of a completely different type from those used in epilepsy may produce a favourable response.

Drop attacks

These affect only middle-aged women, and then often only for a year or two. The story is striking. The woman complains that, while walking along, she suddenly finds that her legs have given way. She may land on her knees or pitch forward on her face. In either case she is always adamant that she is fully aware of what is happening, and equally adamant that she does not trip. The condition is variously assumed to be due to some weakness of the thigh muscles, or to a disturbance of blood flow in the brain-stem, interfering with postural reflexes. Whatever the mechanism, neurologists are confident that there is no association with epilepsy.

Jumping legs (myoclonic jerks; hypnic jerks)

About 80 per cent of the adult population, at some time in their lives, are conscious of a sudden jerk of one or other leg, usually in the twilight stage of drifting off to sleep. The jerk is associated with, or may cause, a sudden arousal. Some people have a great number of jerks, so many that their spouse, being bruised by the kicks, will refuse to share a bed with them. These jerks must represent some sort of paroxysmal discharge of nerve cells, not necessarily in the brain. They are therefore in this way close to epilepsy, but are not so regarded because of their near universality in the population, and their lack of association with frank epileptic seizures. Specifically, there is no relationship between these jerks and the morning myoclonic jerks associated with typical absence or tonic–clonic seizures (p. 13).

Vertigo

Doctors are careful to distinguish true vertigo—a perception of dysequilibrium of the body in its relation to space—from non-specific feelings in the head such as 'dizziness' or 'muzziness' which are so often associated with anxiety and depression. True vertigo is rarely a symptom of a partial seizure in a temporal lobe. Far more common is vertigo due to a disorder of the balancing organ—the labyrinth—lying within the inner ear. The labyrinth may malfunction in an episodic way in both children and adults. In young children the distinction between paroxysmal vertigo and partial seizures may not be easy, as in both the child is frightened, and may either hold on to his mother or fall. The distinction rests on the absence of amnesia or confusion after the attack of benign paroxysmal vertigo, and the presence of abnormal tests of labyrinthine function.

Rigors

Occasionally the shivering associated with high fever, particularly frequent in infections of the urinary tract, may be confused with a convulsion.

Night terrors

These episodes are common in children between the ages of 5 and 10 years and frequently worry parents. Typically a child who has been in bed, asleep for 1–3 hours will waken suddenly, screaming. The child will be sitting up in bed, wide-eyed and unresponsive; they cannot be comforted. Within a minute or so, the child will lie down, turn over, and go back to sleep. There is no memory or recollection of the event the next morning. Reassurance (of the parents) is all that is required.

Rage attacks/outbursts of temper

Bizarre, semi-purposeful behaviour and confusion may rarely be part of a complex partial seizure arising from a temporal lobe. However, violent behaviour or uncontrolled rage are almost never a type of epileptic seizure. They are usually provoked by someone or something, even though the cause may be trivial.

Tics, habits, and ritualistic movements

Tics in children usually involve the upper part of the face—screwing up the eyes, or rapid blinking. More complex habits such as grunting, and brushing the hair away from the eyes are common in children, and seldom confused with seizures. Sometimes, however, children indulge in strange patterns of movement which they apparently find pleasurable, and which they stop immediately on reprimand. Sometimes infants and toddlers will rock backwards and forwards squeezing their thighs together in a manner which seems to be masturbatory.

Colic

Colic or 'wind' is a common symptom in babies and young infants, and is usually easily recognized and diagnosed. However, occasionally infantile spasms (West's syndrome), may be mistaken for colic or some other type of pain, which can lead to a delay in the diagnosis of this type of epilepsy.

Overbreathing

Breathing in and out too fast and too deep is one bodily way in which, like palpitations, anxiety is manifested. This response seems to be particularly common in adolescent girls. If continued for more than a few minutes, excessive carbon dioxide is removed by the lungs from the blood, which becomes correspondingly alkaline. This affects the levels of calcium in the blood, and, in turn, the conduction of nerve impulses and the contraction of muscles. The net effect is that the subject experiences painful tingling in the hands and toes, which become flexed and contracted in a cramped posture. The lack of carbon dioxide also produces a feeling of light-headedness, and the total picture may be confused with a seizure. Treatment is simple and dramatically effective. A paper or polythene bag is placed (temporarily!) over the patient's, nose and mouth, so that she re-breathes her own expired air, rich in carbon dioxide. The body chemistry and clinical state rapidly return to normal.

Simulated seizures

It might seem strange that anyone would wish to pretend to have an epileptic seizure, but in consultant practice this is one of the more common differential diagnoses to be considered. The great majority of such patients have some knowledge of epilepsy—either they have seen a relative with seizures, or more commonly they have had some true seizures themselves. Unless the true and suspect attacks are both seen by an expert, it may be impossible to sort out exactly what is happening. A doctor may be trapped into giving more and more anti-epileptic drugs for seizures which he believes to be out of control. Conversely if he sees one fit which he is quite sure is feigned, he may well wrongly believe all are feigned.

The points which distinguish a true and simulated seizure are the character of the convulsions, which are often not imitated very well. A colleague (David Marsden) has rightly remarked that they are 'intensified by restraint and mollified by inattention'. Incontinence does not distinguish between true and simulated seizures as this can be, and often is, simulated. A normal EEG recorded during a generalized 'seizure' is virtually incontrovertible evidence of simulation. However, the records may be so technically marred by the patient's thrashing around that interpretation is difficult. Combined video and EEG recording is often more helpful.

Psychiatrists, rightly or wrongly, draw a distinction between simulation of disease due to conscious malingering, for example, a man pretending to be sick to avoid conscription to the army, and unconscious hysteria, in which it is alleged that the simulation is the product of the unconscious mind. In each case some potential gain to the patient from the pretence is apparent. The gain in simulating seizures usually is to seek more attention. Rather than lay blame, doctors should regard these events as an indication that patients cannot cope with their life problems, and they should do their best to help and not to blame.

Finally, seizures may occur in a number of other, systemic illnesses or disorders such as hypoglycaemia (low blood sugar) (which may occur in treated diabetes mellitus if too much insulin is given); renal (kidney) failure; hepatic (liver) failure; respiratory (lung) failure; alcohol abuse and its withdrawal; and inborn errors of body metabolism (see p. 28). Finally, the potential effects of prescription or illicit drugs in precipitating seizures must always be considered.

5 Tests in epilepsy

The preceding chapter has made it clear that epilepsy is a clinical diagnosis based on a detailed description of events. There is no single test which can always make, or exclude, a diagnosis of epilepsy. Moreover, as also explained in earlier chapters, epilepsy is not a single condition. There are many different types of epilepsy, and there are many different causes of epilepsy. Investigations may be useful to:

- add weight to, or support the clinical diagnosis of epilepsy;

- help 'classify' the type of epileptic seizure and epilepsy syndrome. This is important in predicting the likely outcome of the epilepsy in a given individual, and the treatment that should be used; and

- help detect or find a cause for the epilepsy.

As we have shown in Table 3.2 (p. 40), no clearly defined cause will be found in about two-thirds of children and adults with epilepsy.

The main investigations which may be used in epilepsy are the electroencephalogram (EEG) and brain imaging techniques, most commonly computerized tomographic scanning (CT scanning) or magnetic resonance imaging (MRI). Other investigations such as X-rays, blood tests, lumbar puncture (spinal tap), or tissue biopsy are much less commonly undertaken.

Electroencephalography (EEG)

The EEG is the principal investigation used in epilepsy. Many patients with epilepsy will have an EEG performed, usually after a clinical diagnosis has been made, and before treatment is started. The EEG detects the brain's electrical activity by sensitive sensors called 'electrodes' which are placed on the scalp; these electrodes detect the normal and abnormal electrical activity of the nerve cells within the brain. Most routine EEGs are recorded with the child or adult awake, but EEGs may be arranged after deprivation of sleep or during sleep (spontaneous or induced by drugs).

All hospitals with neurological or neurosurgical departments and some larger, non-specialized hospitals will have facilities for recording a routine EEG. The procedure is simple and painless and, in the case of a routine EEG takes only about 20–30 minutes to complete. The EEG detects and records the brain's activity; at no time is there any electrical discharge passing from the equipment to the patient. The EEG should not be confused with electroconvulsive therapy or ECT, which is used to treat depressive illnesses, and has *nothing* to do with epilepsy.

The recording technician first measures the patient's head for correct placement of the electrodes, which are then placed according to an international system based on the patient's head size and on measurements taken from the bridge of the nose, and the bony protuberance at the back of the head. Silver electrodes are fastened to the head with a sticky substance called collodion. Alternative electrodes are gauze pads moistened with a salt solution and secured with a rubber cap. Sometimes the patient's scalp is gently rubbed beneath the electrodes to reduce the electrical resistance of the skin which improves the recording. Twelve electrodes are used in small infants, 20 in older children and adults. Wires from each electrode are then connected to a junction box (head-box), connected in turn to the amplifiers of the EEG machine by a cable. After amplification, the EEG machine records the signals on tape or disc, or displays them directly by ink-jets, pens, or laser on to paper which moves at constant speed, usually 3 cm/second. It is this paper with the written waves that is known as 'the EEG' and which is examined and analysed by doctors (Fig. 5.1). The advantage of recording the electrical signals from the different electrodes on to magnetic tape or disc is that they can be recombined in other ways for subsequent more detailed analysis. They can then of course be displayed on paper again at any subsequent time.

During an EEG the child or adult is asked to lie quite still. This is because movement of any part of the body may obscure, or make it difficult to detect the electrical activity of the brain. The technician

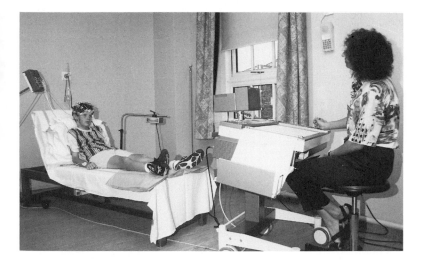

Fig. 5.1 Person having a 'routine' EEG recorded.

also in the course of the recording will ask the patient to open and close the eyes (to look for normal patterns of activity which vary according to whether the eyes are opened or not), to breathe deeply for 3 minutes, and to look at a flashing light. Overbreathing (also called hyperventilation) and the flashing-light test (called photic stimulation) are useful ways of activating or provoking abnormal electrical activity from the brain, and are often important in helping to decide what *type* of seizure (pp. 10–20) or what epilepsy syndrome (pp. 20–2) a person has.

The appearance of the EEG is dependent upon the age of a patient because the brain is developing and maturing rapidly, particularly from birth to 7 or 8 years of age. Generally speaking, a normal adult EEG pattern (Fig. 5.2) is reached by the age of 10–12 years and there is then little change until the age of 60 or 70 years. Doctors who analyse EEGs must have some knowledge and understanding about EEG patterns (normal and abnormal) in infants and children, as well as in adults.

The hallmark or typical EEG finding in a patient with epilepsy between seizures is a 'spike' or 'spike and slow wave' or 'sharp

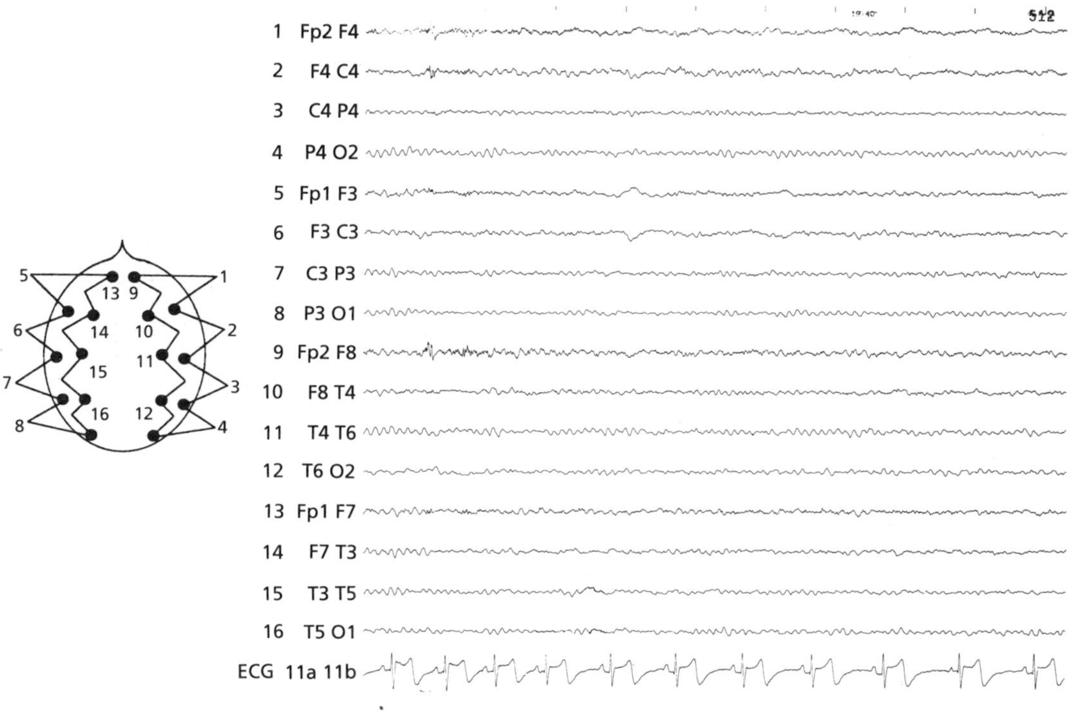

Fig. 5.2 A normal EEG pattern. This pattern is seen from mid-childhood (age 10–12 years) until late adult life (60–70 years).

wave'. A 'spike' is a sudden change in voltage that shows up against the background activities. Examples of focal and generalized EEG abnormalities are shown in Figs 5.3 and 5.4. An example of a very abnormal EEG seen in infants with West syndrome (Chapter 2) is shown in Fig. 5.5. However, even in patients who have epilepsy these abnormalities are not always seen, and this is why the EEG must not be relied upon to make or exclude a diagnosis of epilepsy. The first 20 minute recording of an adult who has had an undoubted tonic–clonic seizure is normal in 40–50 per cent of cases.

For most people with epilepsy, a routine (20–30 minute) EEG is the only necessary test. However, this is only a short period to record the brain's electrical activity, and it is unlikely that a clinical attack or seizure will occur in this time. If more information is required, then other types or systems of EEG recording may be performed.

(a) **EEG after deprivation of sleep**: In this situation a patient is asked to make sure they get only 4–5 hours sleep for two consecutive nights. This encourages the occurrence of seizure discharges. Deprivation of sleep may also lead the patient to drowse or to sleep during the recording, and again this encourages the appearance of abnormal EEG discharge.

(b) **Drug-induced sleep EEG**: A small dose of a sedative drug may encourage the patient to fall asleep during the recording, and again drowsiness and sleep may show abnormalities which may not be present whilst awake.

(c) **Ambulatory EEG monitoring**: This is a technique of recording an EEG for not just 20 or 30 minutes but for up to 24 or even 48 hours. The electrodes (six, eight or 12, rather than the twenty electrodes in a routine EEG) are wired up to a small tape recorder (like a Walkman cassette player) which is strapped to the waist (Fig. 5.6). After this the child or adult can leave the EEG department, go home and carry on their normal activities, and then return to the EEG department after 24 hours to have the tape analysed or the tape replaced. This procedure is more likely, by the length of the recording

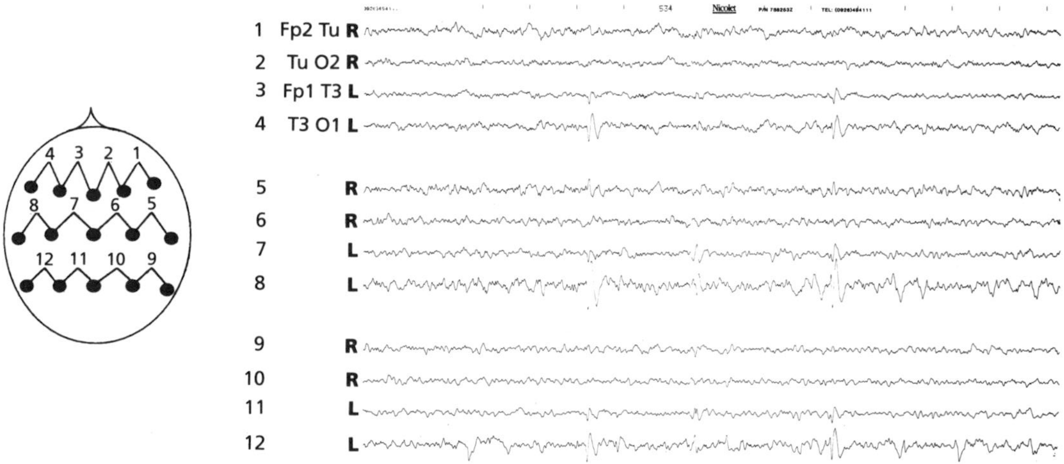

Fig. 5.3 EEG showing a large spike and sharp wave discharge affecting only the left side of the brain. This EEG appearance is seen in patients with partial or location-related (such as temporal lobe) epilepsy.

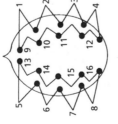

Fig. 5.4 EEG of a young adult showing a brief (two second) 'burst' or discharge of generalized spike and slow wave activity. This EEG appearance is seen in patients with idiopathic or primary generalized epilepsy.

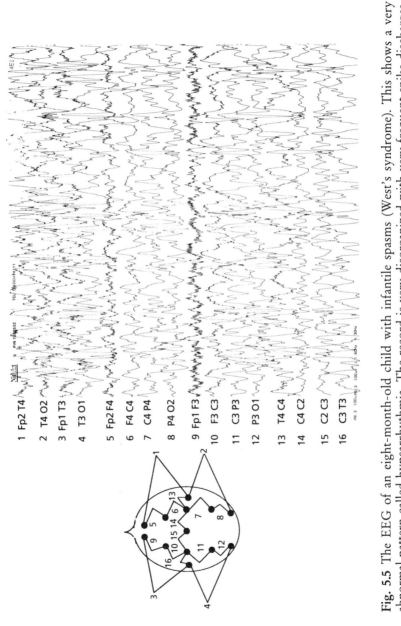

Fig. 5.5 The EEG of an eight-month-old child with infantile spasms (West's syndrome). This shows a very abnormal pattern called hypsarrhythmia. The record is very disorganized with very frequent spike discharges, and no normal brain activity.

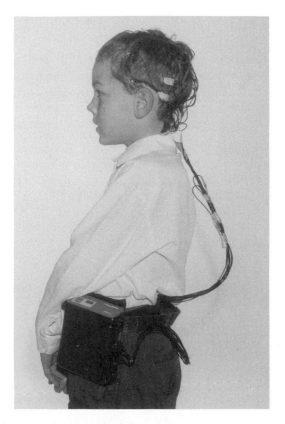

Fig. 5.6 Close-up photograph of the cassette recorder used in an ambulatory EEG recording. The recorder is a little larger than a 'Walkman' recorder and can be strapped to the waist whilst a patient goes around and about doing normal activities. The recorder contains a tape which records the brain's electrical activity over 24 hours. The wires lead up to the electrodes which are attached to the patient's head.

alone, to pick up abnormal electrical activity, and is particularly valuable if the person has a fit or seizure during the 24 hours when the electrical activity is being recorded. The tape can be analysed in a special fast-pace display unit, so the doctor does not have to sit watching the EEG for

24–48 hours! An example of such a recording is shown in Fig. 5.6.

(d) **Depth electrodes**: On rare occasions, special depth electrodes are used. These are fine wires inserted under sterile conditions into areas of the brain thought possibly to be the site of origin of seizure discharge. This is an important test in those patients who are being considered for surgical treatment of their epilepsy (p. 100).

(e) **Video-telemetry**: This is another way of obtaining an EEG over a longer period of time. In this technique the patient has to stay in a room in the hospital for 24 hours or longer. At the same time as the electrical activity is recorded on the EEG, a video camera records the activities of the patient (Figure 5.7). In this way it is possible to replay repeatedly both simultaneous video and EEG

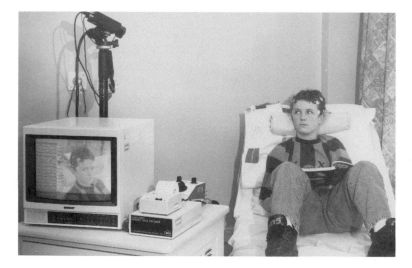

Fig. 5.7 A split-screen video-EEG recording. At the same time as the EEG is being recorded, the patient's behaviour and movements are also recorded by a video-camera. The EEG and the patient are then shown side-by-side on the same television screen. This enables a precise correlation and comparison between the electrical activity of the brain and what is happening clinically to the patient at the same time.

recordings and observe the pattern of the EEG during an attack or seizure. This provides valuable information on the type of epileptic seizure and from where within the brain the seizure may be starting. If no abnormalities are seen on the EEG during an 'attack', then almost certainly the attacks are not epileptic. Video-telemetry is really only of practical benefit if the patient is having frequent attacks, as it is otherwise impractical to keep the patient in hospital attached to expensive equipment on the remote chance that a seizure may occur.

How sensitive is the EEG?

The EEG is often thought to be able either to prove, or to exclude a diagnosis of epilepsy, but this is rarely possible. A single, routine EEG is likely to show any abnormal (and therefore helpful) activity in only about half of those who have had a tonic–clonic (grand mal) seizure. If further, or longer duration EEGs are done, the yield increases. It must therefore be clearly understood that the EEG does not prove, nor disprove the diagnosis of epilepsy. There is one important exception to this, and this is with a type of epilepsy called non-convulsive status epilepticus (p. 104). This may present with bizarre or confused behaviour with semi-purposeful, almost automatic movements. It may be difficult to decide whether this behaviour is epilepsy, but if it is, the EEG helps make the diagnosis

The EEG also is not a good guide to either the activity or prognosis of epilepsy. There is one type of epilepsy, however, in which the EEG is particularly useful—this is typical absence epilepsy (petit mal). In this epilepsy syndrome the frequent seizures may be so brief and subtle that some time may elapse before they are recognized. In children with typical absences, the EEG almost always shows a seizure discharge, which may be induced by hyperventilation, and even more easily after deprivation of sleep.

Table 3.2 shows that for nearly two thirds of cases a cause of epilepsy is not found. The EEG is usually not helpful in identifying a cause. Occasionally, however, the EEG may show marked differences between the two sides of the brain, such as a slow wave discharge arising from one particular area. This suggests the presence of a structural abnormality as the cause of the patient's epilepsy. However, structural abnormalities are best investigated by imaging techniques (brain-scans). These are, after the EEG, the most commonly used investigation in epilepsy.

Brain imaging investigations

The EEG is a *'functional'* investigation, recording the brain's function through normal and abnormal electrical activity. Imaging procedures or brain scans provide information about the brain's *structure*, and revealing normal and abnormal anatomy. Most, if not all patients who have epilepsy need to have at least one EEG, fewer than perhaps 1 in 5 or 1 in 6 patients need to have an imaging investigation. Research is underway to determine who should be scanned.

Two types of imaging techniques are currently available in the developed world; these are the computerized tomographic (CT) brain scan and magnetic resonance imaging (MRI).

The CT scan

This is an abbreviation the computerized axial tomography (CAT) scan. The technique was developed in the 1970s and is a type of X-ray investigation. Tomography is a word dating from earlier X-ray techniques. The patient lies still on a table whilst a rotating X-ray machine takes two-dimensional pictures of the head from many different angles or positions. The information is then processed by a computer to produce pictures (or images) at different levels of the brain. Examples of a normal and abnormal CT scan are shown in Figs 5.9 and 5.10. The test is safe, and other than keeping the head still, there are no particular precautions to be taken. Children may have to be given a sedative drug or short anaesthetic so that they can keep still for the scan. The test takes approximately 15–20 minutes. If an area of interest is seen on the initial images, some contrast (special dye) is injected into a vein in the hand or arm and then the scan repeated. The dye may enhance contrast in areas of interest

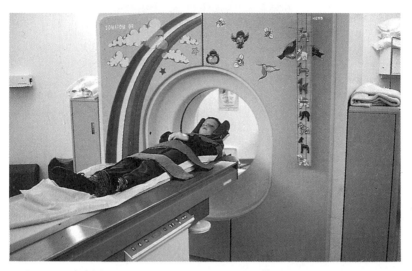

Fig. 5.8 Child having a computerized tomographic (CT) head scan.

and give more detailed information. CT scanning has proved to be very useful in detecting structural abnormalities within the brain, such as strokes, infections, tumours, and congenital malformations which may cause epilepsy. However, only 20–25 per cent of patients with epilepsy referred to special centres will have an abnormal CT scan. Abnormalities on the CT scan in patients who have epilepsy are more likely to be found in the following situations:

- patients whose seizures affect only one side of the body;

- patients whose EEG shows a persistent slow wave abnormality on one side of the brain;

- when epilepsy starts in newborn babies and continues;

- when epilepsy starts in later life; and

- if the patient has abnormal findings on neurological examination, for example, mild weakness down one side of the body, or changes in the reflexes.

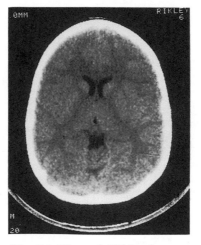

Fig. 5.9 Normal CT head scan.

The MR scan (MRI)

This is often called MRI (magnetic resonance imaging) or nuclear magnetic resonance (NMR). The technique has nothing to do with radiation or X-rays, but records energy given out by atoms as they change their orientation after a brief magnetic pulse. The pictures or images produced have the same general appearance as CT scans, because the information processed by the computer is much the same as (Fig. 5.11 and Fig. 5.12). Again it is necessary for the patient to lie still while the images are being taken.

The procedure is noisier than CT scanning and may, in some patients produce a claustrophobic feeling, as the patient is almost entirely enclosed in a tunnel. MRI usually takes about 25–35 minutes, but may take longer. Occasionally some contrast dye is injected into a vein, as in CT scanning, and then the scan repeated to demonstrate some additional details. Children may find the procedure more uncomfortable than having a CT scan and because of this more often need to have a brief general anaesthetic so that they lie still.

MRI gives a much clearer picture of those areas of the brain (the temporal lobes) which are most often responsible for intractable epilepsy (Fig. 5.12), and so patients who are considered possibly to be suitable for surgery will certainly need an MRI. MRI is also useful for children in whom the epilepsy is thought to be due to a congenital malformation of the brain. Because of its greater costs (at present) MRI is unlikely to replace completely CT scanning, but there is no doubt that the level of detail obtained is far superior with MRI.

Other imaging techniques

Before the development of CT scanning, simple skull X-rays or air-encephalograms (in which the structure of the brain was outlined by injected air) were the only techniques available. These have been superseded entirely. Another technique, angiography, is still used in some patients with epilepsy due to a structural cause. In

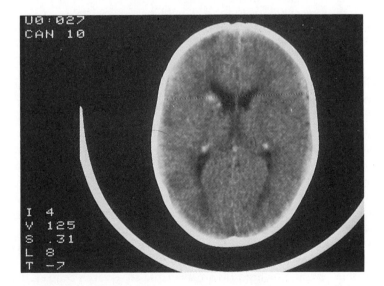

Fig. 5.10 Abnormal CT head scan showing areas of calcification or 'tubers' (the 5 white 'spots') and abnormal brain development in a child with infantile spasms and tuberous sclerosis.

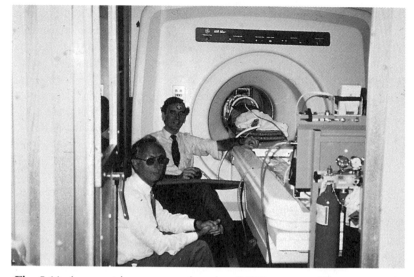

Fig. 5.11 A magnetic resonance imaging (MRI) scanner. The two people facing the camera are an anaesthetist and his assistant who may be needed if a young child needs an anaesthetic to enable him or her to lie still.

this technique, an iodine-containing solution which is opaque to X-rays is injected directly into one or other carotid artery (in the neck), or through a catheter introduced into the brachial (elbow) or femoral (groin) arteries and passed into the region of the carotid. Immediately after the injection, a series of X-ray pictures are taken which outlines the arteries and veins containing the iodine solution. This technique identifies precisely any abnormal blood vessels and may be extremely valuable if surgery is being considered on an angioma (p. 31) or tumour. Advances in MRI mean that the circulation can usually be imaged by special pulse techniques and image processing software, so angiography is likely to be superseded in the near future.

Other imaging techniques are available at research centres. These include positron emission tomography (PET), or single photon emission computerized tomography (SPECT). In these procedures, variations in function in different parts of the brain can be imaged.

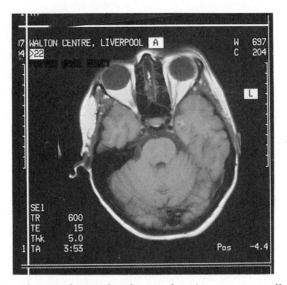

Fig. 5.12 An abnormal MRI head scan showing a very small ring-like tumour in the left temporal lobe of a young adult with repeated partial seizures.

The technique involves injecting a glucose solution, or breathing oxygen, either of which is labelled with a specially marked atom. The oxygen or glucose is taken up and metabolized by different parts of the brain at different rates. The marker atoms attached to the oxygen or glucose allows images to be obtained which may show an area or areas of the brain which take up a lot of oxygen and glucose during a seizure, and which could be an epileptic focus. Between seizures, the same areas are relatively silent. Such studies may help neurologists and neurosurgeons decide on the suitability of a child or adult for epilepsy surgery.

Other tests

Blood tests are seldom informative in patients with epilepsy but may be useful in the early days of life, when chemical abnormalities may precipitate seizures (p. 38). A lumbar puncture may be carried out if an infection such as meningitis or encephalitis is suspected as causing epileptic seizures (p. 37). Occasionally, removal of tissues (biopsy) for microscopic analysis may be helpful in rare causes of epilepsy; the tissues which are biopsied include skin or rectum (as these contain accessible nerve cells) or muscle. The diseases which are being tested for usually have manifestations other than seizures alone.

It is rarely necessary to repeat the EEG or a brain scan in most people with epilepsy. However, there are some exceptions to this general rule. Further EEGs may be helpful if treatment is not as effective as expected, or if, after a period of good seizure control, a patient's seizures become more frequent. Some doctors recommend that an EEG should be repeated before a patient comes off treatment with anticonvulsants, but there is not much evidence that this helps reach a decision. There is rarely any justification for repeating a brain scan. However, if something suspicious is seen on a CT scan, then an MRI scan could be useful in confirming an abnormality, particularly if surgery for the epilepsy is being considered. Clearly if the epilepsy gets markedly worse, or the patient develops new symptoms such as weakness of a limb or develops new neurological signs, then it is essential to investigate the patient again.

In summary, laboratory investigation of seizures has a limited value. An ordinary EEG may rarely improve the certainty of diagnosis, though it more frequently helps ascertain the type of seizure and so the correct choice of anti-epileptic drug. The much more expensive tape-recorded EEGs and video monitoring of seizures do undoubtedly help discriminate between different types of seizures, and between real and simulated attacks.

CT or MR scanning may give a direct visual demonstration of the structural abnormality causing seizures, though this does not often influence management. Simple blood tests and skull X-rays, though cheap to perform, seldom show a relevant abnormality. With this knowledge, the neurologist will often embark upon few if any investigations. His perspective may be that he is faced with a problem that is common in his practice, and that there are well recognized and effective policies for coping with the matter. A good and kind neurologist will recognize that this professional perspective, based on his knowledge and experience, is not that of his patient, who is frightened and bewildered by the onset of events which he does not understand, but which he feels may have important effects on his life and career.

The technical aspects of the neurological consultation—the history, the differential diagnosis, the examination, any necessary investigation, and prescription of anti-epileptic drug—take comparatively little time. Most of the consultation should be spent, in our view, in exploring the person's attitudes and knowledge about epilepsy, and the effect that epilepsy may have on his life, so that practical advice and support can be given. Often this may take more than one consultation. How much of this support should be provided by the neurologist and how much by the family doctor depends upon the personalities of the doctors and the patient, as well as upon the available time. What *is* disastrous for the patient is if each doctor assumes that the other is coping with these aspects.

6   *The treatment of epilepsy*

The treatment of epilepsy begins with making a correct diagnosis—the diagnosis that the events are truly seizures, the diagnosis of the seizure type, and the diagnosis of the epilepsy syndrome (pp. 10–22). This is particularly important in children in whom other non-epileptic, brief disturbances may be confused with and misdiagnosed as epilepsy (pp. 54; 57–8). The drugs which are used to prevent or control epileptic seizures (anti-epileptic drugs; anticonvulsant drugs) may have to be used for some years—even for life—and have side-effects which are occasionally serious. It is therefore important that the diagnosis of epilepsy is correct before these are prescribed.

The reason for taking drugs is to prevent further seizures or fits from occurring. The drugs will only do this if they are taken regularly, and as advised by the doctor. One common reason for people with epilepsy having further attacks is because they either do not want to take, or forget to take their medication regularly.

There are a number of questions to be considered.

Should anti-epileptic medication be given?

A person who has had two or three seizures does not *necessarily* need treatment. For example, an adult who has two or three generalized tonic–clonic seizures (grand mal fits) in a two-week period and who might lose his job if he had a seizure at work requires early treatment, whereas a child who has cerebral palsy and learning difficulties and who had had two partial seizures six months apart does not necessarily require treatment with anti-epileptic drugs. Remember also that there are people whose seizures can be clearly attributed in part to a non-recurring cause. For example, seizures may begin for the first time whilst the person is on an antidepressant drug, such as amitriptyline, which is known to induce seizures in some people. Clearly the drug is not the only factor. Thousands of people take amitriptyline without having seizures. In those who do, the drug presumably acts on those with a low seizure threshold (see p. 3–4). Nevertheless it would seem reasonable to see how such a person gets on without antidepressants, before prescribing anti-epileptic medication. Other precipitating factors, if specific, such as occur in epilepsy induced by television (see p. 44) may be avoided, and make anti-epileptic medication unnecessary.

It is therefore important that each patient is considered as an individual. The choice of whether or not anti-epileptic medication should be used is made in equal partnership between patient (or parent) and doctor. For example, a woman may wish to avoid anti-epileptic medication if planning a pregnancy (see p. 93) even though her chances of further seizures are high.

One common decision that has to be made is whether or not to start anti-epileptic medication after a single seizure in an adult, often for which no clearly defined precipitating factor can be identified. It used to be advised that 'one seizure did not make a diagnosis of epilepsy'. Although true by definition (p. 4), the risk of a second seizure is in adults as high as 78% over the next three years, the risk being its highest in the first few weeks. Recent trials have shown clearly that an anti-epileptic drug given after the first seizure does significantly reduce the chances of a second. Patients should be offered the choice of anti-epileptic medication at this stage, with a clear explanation of the risks of further seizures and the relative drawbacks of medication, even though a number will decide to take their chances.

Which anti-epileptic drug should be used?

Ideally, an anti-epileptic drug will prevent further attacks with no side-effects or at least with side-effects that are acceptable. Whether a side-effect is acceptable or not is largely dependent upon the person taking the medication. The older anti-epileptic drugs such as bromide (never used now) and primidone (still used, though rarely), were associated with many unwanted side-effects, principally drowsiness. The newer anti-epileptic drugs are designed by the pharmaceutical companies to have less prominent side-effects, but, by the very fact that they are newer, we do not yet have much experience of their long term adverse effects.

The principal factors that determine which drug should be given to a patient are the relative effectiveness and safety of the various drugs. We need to choose:

- the anti-epileptic drug which is most effective for the patient's type of seizure and epilepsy syndrome;

- the safest drug which can be used to treat the patient's epilepsy.

We also need to consider:

- how the chosen drug is to be given—that is, in medicine or tablet form, and how many times a day. This is particularly important for children who may need to be prescribed the drug in a flavoured syrup (medicine) as they may not be able to swallow tablets or capsules. School children naturally dislike having to take tablets at school, as this draws unwanted attention. This again may influence the choice of tablet.

The choice of drug for different types of seizure and epilepsy syndromes

Each drug has two names—the generic or chemical name (for example, sodium valproate), and the trade name (for example, Epilim), which is the name given by the maker of the drug. Traditionally but not invariably, generic drugs are written with an initial small letter, and the trade names with an initial capital letter. Doctors may write a prescription using either the generic or trade name. If the generic name is used, the pharmacist in the retail chemist or hospital pharmacy department can provide either the generic or trade drug. If, however, the doctor prescribes the drug using the trade name, then the pharmacist *must* provide the patient with that drug.

Table 6.1 shows the anti-epileptic drugs which are currently available, using generic and trade names, the various preparations of the drug, and the usual adult daily dosage. It is difficult to provide even a guide for children's dosages, as the right dose must be based on the age of the child and their weight. An infant is prescribed a much lower dose of an anti-epileptic drug than a school child.

Table 6.1 Anti-epileptic drugs

Generic name	Trade name	Preparations	Usual adult dosage
Acetazolamide	Diamox	250 mg tablets 250 mg capsules	250–1000 mg/day (taken in one or two divided doses)
Carbamazepine	Tegretol	100, 200, 400 mg tablets 100, 200 mg chew tablets 200, 400 mg Retard tablets (slow release) 100 mg/5 ml sugar-free syrup	400–1000 mg/day (taken in two or three divided doses)
Clobazam	Frisium	10 mg tablets (some hospital pharmacies can make smaller tablets or liquid preparations)	10–30 mg/day (taken in one, two or three divided doses)
Clonazepam	Rivotril Clonopil	0.5, 2.0 mg tablets 1.0 mg/ml ampoule for intravenous use (status epilepticus only)	0.5–4.0 mg/day (taken in one, two or three divided doses)
Diazepam	Valium Diazemuls Stesolid (rectal tube)	2, 5, 10 mg tablets 2 mg/5 ml syrup 10 mg ampoules for intravenous use (status epilepticus) 5 mg or 10 mg Stesolid rectal tubes (status epilepticus)	Not usually taken by mouth

Table 6.1 continued

Generic name	Trade names	Preparations	Usual adult dosage
Ethosuximide	Zarontin Emeside	250 mg capsules 250 mg/5 ml syrup (orange or blackcurrant flavoured)	500–2000 mg/day (taken in two or three divided doses)
Gabapentin	Neurontin	100, 300, 400 mg capsules	900–2400 mg/day (taken in three divided doses)
Lamotrigine	Lamictal	25, 50, 100 mg tablets 5, 25, and 100 mg chewable or dispersable tablets	100–200 **mg/day** in patients receiving sodium valproate. 200–400 **mg/day** in patients *not* receiving sodium valproate (taken in two divided doses)
Nitrazepam	Mogadon	5 mg tablets 2.5 mg/5 ml suspension	10–20 mg/day (taken in one or two divided doses)
Phenobarbitone	Gardenal Luminal Phenobarbitol	15, 30, 60, 100 mg tabs. 30 mg/10 ml syrup	60–200 mg/day (taken in two or three divided doses)

Table 6.1 continued

Generic name	Trade names	Preparations	Usual adult dosage
Phenytoin	Epanutin Dilantin	25, 50, 100, 300 mg caps. 50 mg chewable tablets (Infatabs) 60 mg/10 ml suspension	200–600 mg/day (taken in two or three divided doses)
Primidone	Mysoline	250 mg tablets 250 mg/5 ml liquid suspension	500–1500 mg/day (taken in two or three divided doses)
Sodium valproate	Epilim Depakine Depomide	100 mg crushable tablets 200, 500 mg tablets 200 mg/5 ml syrup 200 mg/5 ml sugar-free liquid 150, 300, 500 mg capsules 200, 300, 500 mg Chrono (slow release) tablets	600–3000 mg/day (taken in two, or rarely three doses)
Vigabatrin	Sabril	500 mg tablets 500 mg/sachet as powder	1000–3000 mg/day (taken in two divided doses)

Table 6.2 shows the generic name of the drug, the types of epilepsy or seizures which each drug is used to treat, and the side-effects that may be associated with the drugs.

Tables 6.1 and 6.2 describe all the common anti-epileptic drugs which may be given by mouth. There are a number of other drugs which are used only in status epilepticus (p. 104), when they are then given by either an injection into a vein (intravenous route) or by administering a special solution into the rectum. These drugs include chlormethiazole (Heminevrin), lignocaine (Xylocard), lorazepam (Ativan), paraldehyde (no trade name). Diazepam (Valium) is probably the drug most frequently employed in the UK.

Chlormethiazole is frequently used in status epilepticus associated with excessive alcohol consumption or in alcohol withdrawal seizures. Paraldehyde is frequently used in children (given intramuscularly or preferably into the rectum). Although an effective drug, it has a strong and characteristic smell. Lorazepam and lignocaine are more commonly used in North America than in the UK.

Two other drugs are frequently used in children, particularly in young children who have myoclonic seizures or infantile spasms (p. 18). These drugs are prednisolone, (Prednesol, Deltacortril) which is given by mouth, and ACTH (which stands for adrenocorticotrophic hormone (Synacthen) which is given by intramuscular injection. Both these drugs have potential adverse effects common to all cortisone-like drugs, such as raising the blood pressure and blood sugar and increasing the risk of developing severe infections. Because of these possible side-effects, other drugs are now being used to treat infantile spasms in young children, including vigabatrin and sodium valproate.

The side-effects of the anti-epileptic drugs

The main side-effects of all the anti-epileptic drugs are summarized in Table 6.2. Generally, there are potentially three types of side-effects which may be associated with any drug, including anti-epileptic drugs.

Allergic or hypersensitive (idiosyncratic) side-effects   These are

Table 6.2

Generic name	Epilepsy/seizure types	Adverse side-effects
Acetazolamide	'Add-on'* in partial or focal epilepsies, and in catamenial epilepsy (seizures related to menstruation)	Nausea, vomiting, pins and needles/ tingling when used in high doses
Carbamazepine	Drug of choice in complex partial seizures, simple partial seizures, generalized tonic–clonic seizures	Dose-related: nausea, double vision, unsteadiness; allergic: rash, reduced, white blood cell count, increased appetite (rarely) no obvious effect on concentration, memory, or behaviour
Clobazam	'Add-on' in tonic–clonic, myoclonic and partial epilepsies and seizures. Effective in catamenial epilepsy (menstrual seizures).	Dose-related: drowsiness and lethargy. With time the drug loses its effect, despite increasing doses (called 'tolerance').
Clonazepam	Drug of second or third choice in myoclonic seizures. Effective as 'add-on' therapy in tonic–clonic and absence seizures. May be used in status epilepticus.	Dose-related: drowsiness, lethargy, drooling, and hyperactive behaviour in children. With time the drug loses its effect. May cause inflammation of veins.
Diazepam	Drug of choice in status epilepticus (given rectally or intravenously). Rarely used on a regular basis in tablet form.	Dose-related; as with clonazepam. May cause inflammation of veins.

* By 'add-on' we mean that the drug is a second or third line drug which may give a useful additional effect to a first choice such as carbamazepine.

Table 6.2 continued

Generic name	Epilepsy/seizure types	Adverse side-effects
Ethosuximide	Drug of first or second choice for typical absence seizures (petit mal epilepsy). May be effective in myoclonic seizures. Not effective for generalized tonic–clonic seizures.	Dose-related: drowsiness, nausea, vomiting, headache and 'irritability'. Allergic: rashes.
Gabapentin	'Add-on' therapy in partial or focal seizures/epilepsies	Dose-related: drowsiness, lethargy, nausea
Lamotrigine	'Add-on', and, in patients over 12 years of age, mono-therapy in generalized tonic–clonic epilepsy/seizures (possible second choice after sodium valproate). Effective in absences with myoclonic seizures and in partial/focal seizures.	Dose-related; sedation, unsteadiness and possibly worsening of seizures. allergic; rash—this may occur in up to 10% of patients, particularly if sodium valproate is being taken at the same time. To avoid this rash, the drug must be introduced very gradually.
Nitrazepam	Occasionally used for myoclonic and partial seizures (most frequently used in children for infantile spasms).	Dose-related: drowsiness, lethargy, and irritability. Loses its effect fairly quickly (tolerance).

Table 6.2 continued

Generic name	Epilepsy/seizure types	Adverse side-effects
Phenobarbitone	Effective in generalized tonic–clonic, myoclonic and partial seizures. Not a preferred drug. Effective in status epilepticus.	Dose-related: drowsiness, lethargy, unsteadiness. Chronic use: tolerance and impairment of concentration, memory slowness in activities. Withdrawal seizures if the drug is discontinued too quickly.
Phenytoin	Drug of second or third choice in generalized tonic–clonic seizures. Effective in partial (focal) and myoclonic seizures. Drug of choice in status epilepticus.	Dose-related: nausea, vomiting, unsteadiness, slurred speech. Allergic: rash, hepatitis (inflammation of the liver), swelling of lymph glands, chronic use: gum swelling, acne, hairiness (face, body), folate deficiency, involuntary movements, rickets
Primidone	Rarely used for generalized tonic–clonic, absence, and myocloric seizures.	Similar to phenobarbitone (because primidone is broken down to phenobarbitone in the body).

Table 6.2 continued

Generic name	Epilepsy/seizure types	Adverse side-effects
Sodium Valproate	Drug of first choice in primary generalized tonic–clonic seizures, typical absence seizures (petit mal), atonic seizures, myoclonic seizures, and photosensitive epilepsy. Effective in partial or focal seizures (second choice after carbamazepine).	Dose-related: tremor, sedation, restlessness, increased appetite. Allergic: stomach irritation, inflammation of the liver (hepatitis), or pancreas. Chronic use: hair loss (usually transient), weight-gain, low platelets in blood (may cause excessive bleeding if cut).
Vigabatrin	'Add-on' therapy in partial/focal seizures with or without secondary generalization. May be effective in children with infantile spasms.	Dose-related: rarely sedation or changes in behaviour, and confusion.

rare and occur usually within one or two weeks of starting the drug. The effects are usually unpredictable, and, once they have occurred, it means that the drug must be stopped and can probably not be used again. The most common side-effect of this type is a widespread, itchy rash. This occurs in about 5 per cent of patients soon after starting on an anti-epileptic drug. The drugs which may cause rashes are carbamazepine, lamotrigine, phenobarbitone, and phenytoin.

Dose-related side-effects   These may be caused by either introducing the drug too quickly or by giving too much. Most of the anti-epileptic drugs can cause such side-effects, which include drowsiness, confusion, unsteadiness, nausea, vomiting, or headache. These effects can be avoided by starting the drug more slowly and they disappear if the dose is reduced. In children and adults who have severe learning difficulties, dose-related side-effects may be difficult to recognize, as these patients may not be able to describe them.

Long term or chronic side-effects   These are side-effects that develop more slowly, over months or years. They are more common in patients taking more than one drug, and often in high doses. Once again, the effects may be more difficult to recognize (by both the patient and doctor), as they tend to develop gradually and do not cause any acute or sudden problem. The older drugs such as phenobarbitone, primidone, and phenytoin are more likely to cause chronic, or long-term, toxicity. The newer anti-epileptic drugs would appear to be safer. However, as already stated, there is relatively little information on these newer drugs, as they have not yet been used for many years.

One of the most common concerns of patients and parents of children who are receiving anti-epileptic drugs is the effect of drugs on school or work performance, memory, mood, and behaviour. Anti-epileptic drugs may cause some initial drowsiness, or changes in mood and behaviour, as the drug is being started, but these effects usually wear off. The older anti-epileptic drugs such as phenobarbitone and phenytoin have been shown to reduce a patient's concentration or attention span and therefore cause an impairment in memory. This in turn can adversely affect learning and the ability to do certain tasks. These problems are less likely to occur with drugs such as carbamazepine, sodium valproate, vigabatrin, and lamotrigine, although it is impossible to guarantee that they have no effect. It is often difficult to determine whether a problem with either learning or behaviour is definitely due to a drug. A number of patients, as well as having epilepsy, may also have learning and behavioural difficulties as another manifestation of the brain problems that are causing epilepsy. A careful analysis of the story often shows that these difficulties appeared *before* any drug treatment was started, and that the drugs are not responsible.

Phenytoin has an unfortunate effect on the gums, which tend to thicken and grow down between the teeth. This can usually be kept at bay by twice daily brushing upwards and downwards with a medium bristle tooth brush. If necessary a dentist can push back the gums or remove the excessive tissue. This overgrowth of gum tissue is reflected in subtle changes in the lips and facial skin, which may become slightly 'fleshy'. Phenytoin and barbiturates predispose to acne of the face and back, and may cause some slight excess of facial hair. These cosmetic effects may be a reason to avoid using these drugs in young people. Sodium valproate, on the other hand, may cause hair to fall from the scalp in a very small number of people. Regrowth of hair usually occurs even without stopping the drug.

There are a number of other side-effects of anti-epileptic drugs. Phenobarbitone seems to affect the shoulder joint in a few people, so that it becomes stiff and painful. In others, changes in the tendons in the hands and connective tissue of the palms leads to a contracture (Dupuytren's contracture) of the hands. Phenytoin may cause an excessive metabolism of the body's vitamin D supplies, which may lead to rickets, in the absence of adequate diet or sunlight (which helps form vitamin D).

Finally, and importantly, there is the issue of the effect of anti-epileptic drugs on the developing baby—a particular concern to women with epilepsy. There is a slight increase in the occurrence of fetal abnormalities of mothers who have epilepsy. From the analysis of a large number of patients, it is clear that much of this increase is due to anti-epileptic drugs, particularly phenobarbitone and phenytoin. Phenytoin produces a number of abnormalities including a characteristic face, a cleft-(hare) lip or palate, very small and under-developed finger and toe nails, heart defects, spina bifida, and learning difficulties. It must be stressed that this does not occur in the babies of all women taking phenytoin in pregnancy. It will occur in only about 5–10 out of every 100 mothers who have epilepsy and are taking phenytoin, but this risk is about two or three times the risk in women who do not have epilepsy. Sodium valproate, and to a lesser extent carbamazepine, may also cause spina bifida, a malformation of the vertebrae and spinal cord. This risk of sodium valproate causing spina bifida is 1–2 per cent. It is important to realize that these malformations arise early in pregnancy—perhaps even before the mother realizes that she is pregnant. For this reason it is wise to discuss pregnancy and anti-epileptic drugs with doctors *before* conception. During the pregnancy the growth and development of the baby can be monitored closely by detailed ultrasound examinations, which will usually detect major heart abnormalities or severe spina bifida.

Finally, it is also important to realize that if a mother has frequent generalized tonic–clonic (grand mal) seizures during pregnancy this may actually cause more harm to the baby than the drugs themselves—either by direct injury to the abdomen as the mother falls, or by the seizure preventing a sufficient oxygen supply in the mother's, and therefore in the baby's, blood. Although both of these circumstances are rare, they may occur, and because of this it is recommended that anti-epileptic drugs are taken during pregnancy, but that the blood levels are closely monitored (see p. 96). However, it must be stressed that the decision must be taken by patient and doctor together in equal partnership.

The issue of side-effects or toxicity is frequently undervalued by doctors. Minimal side-effects (as defined by an individual or parent of a child and not by the doctor) may be acceptable providing seizure control is good. Major side-effects with or without seizure control are usually unacceptable. What may be acceptable to one patient (or family) may be unacceptable to another. The control of seizures in patients with difficult epilepsy may be improved or achieved by doses of drugs that may cause significant adverse effects. In many of these patients a compromise has to be reached, and a narrow line steered between controlling the seizures without producing excessive sedation or loss of other abilities.

How is the anti-epileptic drug to be given?

The most appropriate drug for the patient's seizure type or epilepsy syndrome must be given in the preparation which is most acceptable to the patient. For adult patients this will usually be in tablet or capsule form, for young children it will be a flavoured liquid or syrup (preferably sugar-free in order to avoid bringing on tooth decay). The drug should be started gradually, and introduced over a 10–14 day period. Most drugs (in whichever preparation) need to be given twice, or occasionally, three times a day in order to maintain as steady a state as possible in the blood. Because phenobarbitone and phenytoin are so slowly broken down in the body, these drugs can be given only once a day. When given two or three times a day, each dose should be more or less the same in order to avoid any dose-related side-effects, which are more likely if one large dose is given. Dose-related side-effects may be avoided by the use of sustained or 'controlled-release' preparations. Sustained or controlled-release means that the drug is released more slowly into the bloodstream from the small bowel. This reduces the chance of acute dose-related side-effects such as unsteadiness, vomiting, sedation, double vision, or tremor. Examples of such preparations are Tegretol Retard and Epilim Chrono.

As far as possible only one anti-epileptic drug should be prescribed at a time (monotherapy). Most patients, both children and adults, will have their epilepsy controlled by a single drug. The remainder, perhaps 30 per cent of these patients, will need to take two or even (very rarely), three anti-epileptic drugs (polytherapy). The choice of a second drug again depends upon the type of seizure and known side-effects of the drugs, and any interaction between the two. As an example, in typical absence epilepsy (petit mal), the first choice drug would be sodium valproate. If seizures were not fully controlled on this drug, the first step would be to consider whether the dose was adequate. Only then would a second choice drug be added—probably ethosuximide or lamotrigine.

Drug interactions—which other drugs can be safely taken with anti-epileptic drugs?

Patients with epilepsy experience other illnesses or infections like anyone else, and have to take additional drugs to treat them. This includes taking antibiotics for infections, analgesics for pain relief (for example, headaches), treatment for asthma. Many women will also want to use the contraceptive pill. Most drugs can be taken safely with all the anti-epileptic drugs, however, there are one or two important exceptions:

- carbamazepine, phenytoin, and phenobarbitone interfere with the effectiveness of the oral contraceptive pill, leading to less reliable contraception. Sodium valproate does *not* appear to have this effect.

- sodium valproate and aspirin may interact and cause excessive bleeding after a cut or injury

- carbamazepine and theophylline (used in asthma)—may reduce the effectiveness of carbamazepine, leading to increased seizures.

It is important that people with epilepsy tell their doctor about any other drugs that they are taking. Interactions between the drugs may provide an explanation for an increase in seizure frequency or status epilepticus (p. 103).

When patients are taking more than one anti-epileptic drug, this increases the risk of developing unpleasant side-effects, particularly if phenytoin is one of the drugs. Any changes in the doses of the two drugs must be made gradually and the patient may need to have blood levels of the drugs measured at intervals.

When should another anti-epileptic drug be given?

As mentioned above, the first choice drug should be used alone (monotherapy) and in the lowest dose to control seizures without producing any unacceptable side-effects. If the initial control of seizures is less than complete, then the dose of that drug should be increased gradually until either complete control is achieved, or side-effects develop. If unacceptable side-effects occur before control is reached, then there are two alternatives: either a different drug can be used to replace the first drug, or an additional drug can be added to the first drug. Which alternative is chosen depends on the individual patient and also on the doctor. If there has been some reasonable control with the first drug, it is our practice to add the next most appropriate anti-epileptic drug without withdrawing the first drug. If complete seizure control is then achieved, we will attempt to withdraw the first drug after a period of two to three months free from seizures. If the initial drug has been ineffective we would simultaneously replace the first drug with the second. In some children and adults, therapy with two anti-epileptic drugs is justified, as this may result in further significant (even complete) control in an additional 5 per cent to 10 per cent of children. It is unlikely that polytherapy with three drugs will result in any further control, and there is certainly an increased risk and frequency of side-effects and toxicity due to interactions between this many drugs.

How is treatment monitored—including 'blood levels' of drugs?

Any patient's response to treatment with anti-epileptic drugs is based first on whether the seizures have reduced in frequency or stopped completely, and secondly whether there have been any side-effects. If a patient has good seizure control but unacceptable side-effects then the dose of the drug should be reduced slightly in the expectation that seizure control will continue, but the adverse effects become less prominent. If the patient has some, but not complete seizure control and no side-effects, then the dose is increased. Therefore, a patient is receiving the correct dose of the drug when the seizures have stopped and there are no side-effects. In the past, doctors used to emphasize the importance of blood tests to measure the amount of drug in the blood (called 'therapeutic blood level monitoring'). This is because there is some relationship between the blood level of the drug and its therapeutic and toxic effects. That is to say, there are blood levels of anti-epileptic drugs below which therapeutic effects do not occur (the drug is unlikely to be effective), and above which no further benefit is achieved without causing toxicity. However, the 'lowest' and 'highest' levels in the blood are only approximate guidelines. For an individual patient the optimal or satisfactory blood level may lie outside these ranges. Up to 50 per cent of patients may be controlled with blood levels well below the lower limit of the range previously considered to be therapeutic, and up to 15–20 per cent of patients may be controlled with no side-effects with blood levels that are higher than the upper limit.

There are many factors which affect the blood levels of anti-epileptic drugs, including the chemical structure of the drug and how it is carried in the blood (usually attached to proteins); the age and sex of the patient; an individual's metabolism of the drug (by either the kidney or liver, and whether there is any disease of these organs); and how regularly and reliably the drug is taken. Because of all these factors, the lack of a clear correlation between blood levels and effectiveness or toxicity, and the fact that a blood test may be distressing (particularly for children), doctors are now less inclined to monitor anti-epileptic drug blood levels. However, there are certain situations where measuring blood levels may be important, including:

- where there is the possibility of the patient not taking the drug as prescribed. This is one of the common reasons for poor seizure control. Measuring the blood level of the drug will go some way to confirm or exclude this possibility;

- if the patient presents in status epilepticus, that is, in a prolonged fit;

- if the patient has severe learning difficulties and is not able to tell the doctor of side-effects;

- if the patient is taking phenytoin, particularly with another anti-epileptic drug. This is because the metabolism of phenytoin is different from all other anti-epileptic drugs. A small change in dosage, either up or down, may respectively result in toxicity or loss of control of seizures.

- special situations, including pregnancy, or when there is a disorder of the kidney or liver. This is because these three situations may significantly affect how the drug is metabolized in the body.

How to help children and adults take their drugs regularly

If a drug is to be taken reliably and regularly, a patient must be informed fully about that drug. A plan of the proposed management and possible side-effects of the anti-epileptic drug must be discussed with the patient (or family) at diagnosis and at the outset of treatment. In the children's seizure clinic at the Royal Liverpool Children's Hospital (Alder Hey) and at St. Bartholomew's Hospital, families are provided with a drug information sheet with written details about the drug. Included is information about:

- its preparation (e.g. tablet, capsule, or liquid);

- the method of administration;

- the dosage regime;

- its possible interactions with drugs bought over the counter in chemist's shops as well as with other prescribed drugs; and

- its side-effects.

Advice is also given regarding what to do about doses which are forgotten, missed, or vomited.

Written information is in addition to, rather than a substitute for, oral advice. Patients often do not remember, or may misunderstand, much of what is said to them by doctors in a busy hospital clinic or surgery. This is particularly relevant with regard to adverse events or side-effects. Unexpected side-effects may distress or annoy patients (and their families) and thus adversely affect whether they will continue to take the drug, with its potential benefits. Patients should also be warned that different, or additional drugs may be needed depending on the specific epilepsy syndrome and their initial response to treatment. Well-informed patients and families are more likely to use their drugs with discretion and obtain the benefits which modern drugs can offer.

What else may be used to treat epilepsy?

The use of anti-epileptic drugs is clearly the principal method of treating epilepsy. In those situations where a specific cause for the seizures has been found, then other treatments may be necessary. This will include antibiotics if the cause is meningitis or a cerebral abscess, antiviral drugs for certain types of encephalitis caused by viruses, supplementation of the diet with vitamins or other substances in those rare disorders where there may be a deficiency, and the use of surgery to remove cysts, tumours, or abnormal areas of the brain. Counselling and other specific psychological programmes designed to help modify behaviour may also be required for certain people, including those who drink alcohol to excess, or who use illicit drugs.

Dietary manipulation

There have been a number of attempts to control epileptic seizures by modifying the diet. This arose from the observation many years ago that fasting or starvation seemed to be associated with a reduction in the frequency of seizures. In the fasting state, normal metabolism is altered with the appearance of substances in the blood and urine, called ketones. It is not known how or why ketones are linked with seizure control. Of course, there may be no direct relationship between the two, and the occurrence of the two together may be coincidental. A diet was discovered which produced ketones, but without the child having to be starved. The diet is very rich in fat and oils, which makes it rather unpalatable. Because 70 per cent of the diet is in this fat form (the remaining 30 per cent coming from protein and carbohydrate), extra vitamins and minerals (such as calcium and magnesium) must be given. In spite of all the fat and oil eaten in this diet, there is no change in the blood level of cholesterol which is responsible for causing coronary heart disease. The main disadvantages with this diet are the unpalatability, often unpleasant diarrhoea, and the fact that the diet must be strictly followed. Its use is usually restricted to infants and children with very severe epilepsy (often with the Lennox–Gastaut syndrome). Unfortunately its success is limited and usually short-lived.

A rarely used and less successful diet is called the oligoantigenic diet. This entails trying to identify those substances in the diet which may cause an increase in epileptic seizures, and then to exclude them from the diet.

There are few, extremely rare conditions, where the epilepsy is caused by an 'inborn error of metabolism'. This means that either the body is missing, or is unable to use, a particular substance—usually a vitamin or enzyme, and, as a result the person develops epilepsy, and often other problems (for example, skin rashes, loss of hair, failure to grow). If the missing substance is then given in large doses, then the epilepsy may stop. An example of this is a condition called pyridoxine (vitamin B6)-dependent seizures, which usually begins by affecting babies or infants in the first few days or weeks of life.

Surgery

The surgical treatment of epilepsy is becoming increasingly useful, particularly when the seizures are not controlled by anti-epileptic drugs. However, surgery must only be undertaken after a careful detailed assessment of the patient. This, and the operation, should only be carried out in recognized specialist centres. This is because both the assessment of the patient, and the operation itself involve expert and sophisticated procedures—and clearly surgery is an irreversible treatment.

Surgical treatment depends on two main principles or ideas. The first is that a local abnormal area of brain can be entirely removed, leaving behind only healthy, normal brain. The second is that the spread of the seizure discharge (to involve other parts of the brain as is illustrated in Fig. 2.1), can be prevented by cutting the nerve fibres which cause the discharge. Penfield and Rasmussen, two Canadian neurosurgeons, were the pioneers of surgery for epilepsy and much of the surgical assessment and treatment of patients today is based on their early work. One of the most important questions that must be answered before surgery can be considered is from where precisely within the brain do the seizures originate. When the cause is a tumour or cyst, then this is relatively easy, but frequently the cause is an area of brain that developed abnormally in fetal life. The identification of the abnormal part of the brain relies upon magnetic resonance imaging, and the use of special electrodes to try and record or 'capture' the epileptic discharge. The scalp electrodes (used in a routine EEG) are not usually sensitive enough for this task, and so other electrodes, called depth electrodes, are frequently used. They are also called 'sphenoidal' or 'foramen ovale' electrodes because this describes how they are placed close to the brain. Electrodes may even have to be placed directly on the surface of the brain, or, as fine silver needles, within its substance. Because these special electrodes are in very close contact with the brain, there is a much greater chance that they will pick up the epileptic discharge.

As well as these assessments, people being considered for surgery may also need detailed psychological evaluation, specifically to try and identify which side of the brain is responsible for language and memory, so that these areas are not damaged during the operation. Consideration must also be given to avoid operating in those parts of the brain responsible for movement—it would be unacceptable to stop the seizures at the expense of causing a paralysis on one side of the body (hemiplegia), which might result in losing the ability to walk or write.

Before a patient is considered for surgical treatment of their epilepsy, it must have been shown that the patient's seizures could not be adequately controlled using anti-epileptic drugs. For how long a patient should not have been controlled is dependent on individual circumstances. It is unwise to operate too early, as the epilepsy might remit (stop) spontaneously, although this is unlikely in the difficult epilepsies. However, if surgery is delayed for too long, then this may limit the potential success of the operation, either because the patient has suffered irreversible educational and social consequences of repeated seizures, or because other parts of the brain which were previously normal may have developed abnormal foci of electrical activity as a result of the continuing activity of the primary focus. Generally speaking most patients with difficult, drug-resistant epilepsy are being considered for surgery too late; surgery can safely be undertaken in children—even young infants. Most specialists would now consider that if acceptable seizure control has not been achieved using optimal doses of anti-epileptic drugs after one to two years, then surgery should be considered as the next step in a patient's treatment. It has been estimated that many patients in the UK might currently benefit from surgery, but only about 200 operations per year are at present being performed.

There are four types of surgical procedure that are currently undertaken:

• removing a large, identifiable lesion such as a tumour or cyst.

• removing an entire cerebral hemisphere. This is done when the whole of one side of the brain is abnormal, this being associated with a hemiplegia (weakness down one side of the body). The operation sounds dramatic, but is often successful leading to a complete resolution of seizures and, frequently, an improvement in the hemiplegia. Hemispherectomy is particularly useful in children with the Sturge–Weber syndrome (p. 31).

• removing a small or large lesion which has been identified on the basis of detailed specialized EEG recording and imaging. This procedure is the one frequently used in temporal lobe epilepsy, where different parts and amounts of the temporal lobe are removed. Advances in imaging have led to the identification of subtle structural abnormalities in the temporal lobes, which are responsible for seizures.

• carrying out a disconnection procedure; this is to try and separate the focus (site of abnormal electrical activity) of origin of the seizure from other parts of the brain, by cutting the nerve fibres which allow the epileptic discharge to spread. Operations attempted have included division (cutting) of the corpus callosum. This is a large band of fibres which transmits electrical information from one hemisphere to another. A more sophisticated, technically difficult procedure (called subpial transection) appears to be more successful.

Overall, the results of epilepsy surgery are encouraging, as many as 60–70 per cent of people who have operations for epilepsy have no further seizures, whilst another 10–20 per cent are much improved. Patients undergoing a hemispherectomy or temporal lobectomy do better than patients who have a corpus callosotomy. For some patients who have had to live with uncontrolled seizures for many years, a cure of their epilepsy following surgery may come as something of a 'shock', requiring a major adjustment in their lives. These patients need careful and expert support and counselling.

It must be emphasized again that patients must be assessed carefully in specialist centres before undergoing surgical treatment of their epilepsy. No one person can have a guarantee that their seizures will stop.

Other treatments

These include hypnosis, aromatherapy, bio-feedback, and acupuncture. The success of these techniques, for which there is little or no scientific evidence of effectiveness, is variable and limited. However, patients may find them of value in giving a sense of control over their bodies and their lives. A new procedure, long-term stimulation of the vagus nerve is at present being evaluated.

General principles

The treatment of epilepsy extends far beyond the prescription of anti-epileptic medication. It is, of course, important to correctly identify the type of epilepsy and to prescribe the most appropriate anti-epileptic drug to obtain the best possible control of seizures without side-effects. However, for many patients and their families, social and psychological factors far outweigh the problem of preventing or controlling the seizures. Help may best be given through a multi-disciplinary approach, preferably within a specialist clinic with advice from a number of different specialists, including nurses, psychologists, and psychiatrists. Many patients get practical help and support from voluntary associations such as the British Epilepsy Association, and patients should be informed of their address and telephone number. A list of associations and their addresses appears in the Appendix.

Treatment of special situations

Status epilepticus

Occasionally, a single, generalized tonic–clonic (grand mal) or generalized absence (petit mal) seizure may be prolonged (lasting

more than 30 minutes) or the seizures may follow each other in
rapid succession without full recovery between each one. When
this happens, it is called status epilepticus. There are a number of
different types of status epilepticus, the most common are:

convulsive status   — prolonged tonic–clonic seizure
                                     — repeated myoclonic seizures

non-convulsive status   — prolonged absence seizure
(non-convulsive means that   — prolonged complex partial seizure
there are no jerks or abnormal
movements)

epilepsia partialis continua   — continuous twitching of
                                       one arm/leg
(this is rare)   or one side of the face, or both.

The EEG is not usually helpful in convulsive status, but may be
extremely valuable in non-convulsive status. In this type of status, the
diagnosis of epilepsy may not be immediately obvious. The patients
may just appear confused or bewildered, with some inappropriate
behaviour. An EEG recorded at this time will confirm the diagnosis.

Convulsive status epilepticus is a medical emergency which
requires prompt treatment. When a convulsion is prolonged, or
a patient does not recover fully between seizures there is a danger
that a lack of an adequate oxygen supply to the brain may cause
brain damage. There is also the risk of vomiting with aspiration of
the vomit into the lungs. Although rare, patients may die in status
epilepticus.

The longer the patient has been in status epilepticus, the harder
it is to stop it.

Treatment consists of giving a fast-acting anti-epileptic drug as
quickly as possible. This is usually given into a vein, or if this is
difficult (which may be the case in young children), into the rectum.
The most commonly used drug is diazepam (also called Valium,
Diazemuls, or in a rectal tube preparation, Stesolid). Stesolid may
be given by parents at home. This is useful as it means that treatment
can be given early and before waiting for a doctor to arrive, or for
the child to be taken to hospital. Other drugs that are sometimes
used include lorazepam (Ativan), chlormethiazole (Heminevrin),

and paraldehyde. This drug is usually given via the rectum but may, rarely be administered as an intramuscular injection into the buttocks. Paraldehyde is a very effective anticonvulsant but its main disadvantage is its unpleasant smell.

If the first dose of either diazepam, lorazepam, or paraldehyde does not terminate the status, then a second dose may be given. If this is not successful then the patient must be treated more urgently, and admitted to the intensive care unit. This is because the suppression of the seizure may require such considerable amounts of drugs that normal breathing may also be suppressed. In this situation, patients may require ventilator-assisted respiration, and intensive nursing. The longer-acting drugs which are most commonly used include phenytoin and phenobarbitone. They are usually given by a 'drip' intravenously to ensure that they work quickly. As the seizure comes under control, drugs can be given again by mouth.

Once the patient has recovered and is stable, any factors which may have caused the status epilepticus must be identified to try and prevent a recurrence. In many situations, this will involve a review of the usual oral anti-epileptic medication, and ensuring that patients take their medication regularly.

Infantile spasms

The treatment of infantile spasms is unlike that of other epilepsies. Treatment usually consists of giving a steroid, either by intramuscular injection, or by mouth. The drug which is given by injection is called ACTH (adrenocorticotrophic hormone), and by mouth, prednisolone. The injections are usually given once (rarely twice) a day for two weeks until the spasms have stopped, and then every other day, and eventually just once a week. Only about one half to two-thirds of children will respond to ACTH or prednisolone, and a number of these children will relapse (have further spasms) once the medication is discontinued. Unfortunately, these medications may be associated with serious side-effects, and therefore the children must be monitored very closely. Other drugs which may be useful in treating spasms include: sodium valproate (Epilim) and nitrazepam (Mogadon). More recently, one of the newer anti-epileptic drugs, vigabatrin (Sabril) is appearing to be successful in treating spasms, particularly if the cause is tuberous sclerosis or as a result of earlier meningitis/encephalitis. This drug seems to be safer, with less serious side-effects, than the steroid drugs. It may soon become the 'first choice' drug in the treatment of infantile spasms. One of us already uses vigabatrin to treat every child who has infantile spasms, irrespective of the cause because it appears to have so few side-effects.

7 The long-term outlook

Many patients, family doctors, and even paediatricians and neurologists, are remarkably pessimistic about the likelihood of seizures stopping—a pessimism which is unjustified by the facts. Pessimism stems from hospital experience. In the past, when neurologists were fewer on the ground, they tended to see only those with the worst epilepsy with the worst prognosis. As they taught the future family doctors, these too were infected with the same pessimism.

What are the facts? The first point to define is what we mean by remission or cessation of seizures. Epilepsy was defined on p. 4 as a 'continuing tendency to epileptic seizures'. A liability to have a seizure, or a lower than average epileptic threshold (p. 29), probably does continue throughout life as part of one's genetic inheritance. A man aged 30, who had some seizures in his teens, cannot be said to be entirely free from the risk of a further seizure right until the end of his life—but his risk may have declined so that it has become, at the age of 30, only a little greater than that of the general population. Regardless of this philosophical discussion, what a person with epilepsy wants to know is whether, for all practical purposes, the seizures will stop. A remission, therefore, can be defined as a certain period free from seizures. The good evidence about the chances of achieving a good long time free from seizures, and, for all practical purposes, permanent freedom, comes from the work in Olmstead county, USA, to which we have already referred in Chapter 2. Figure 7.1 is redrawn from this study. The upright line on the graph indicates the cumulative chance of achieving a remission of at least five years. It can be seen that, at one year after diagnosis, 42 per cent of the patients had entered a seizure-free period that was to extend for at least five years. The probability of being in remission currently (five years or more and continuing), was 61 per cent at 10 years after diagnosis and 70 per cent at 20 years after diagnosis. The difference between the top two curves represents the small numbers of patients who have one long remission of at least five years with subsequent relapse. The bottom curve refers to those patients in remission without drugs. Data from the National General Practice Study on Epilepsy is very similar. At six years after a seizure of any type (excluding acute symptomatic and single seizures) 92 per cent of people had achieved a remission lasting at least one year, 67 per cent lasting at least three years, and 42 per cent a remission lasting at least five years—this last figure being identical to that from Olmstead County. This latter study has followed up people for rather longer than the UK study, and 20 years after the diagnosis of epilepsy, about 30 per cent of patients continued to have seizures, 20 per cent continued to take anticonvulsant medication but had been free from seizures for at least five years, and about 50 per cent had been free from seizures without anti-epileptic medication for at least five years.

Long-term outlook in children

It is difficult, if not impossible to provide an overall prognosis for epilepsy in children, because of the differing ages of onset, different epilepsy syndromes, differing causes of epilepsy, and the varying response to treatment.

However, certain factors are known to be associated with a poor outcome, with seizures unresponsive or only partly responsive to treatment. These factors include:

- epilepsy that starts before the age of two or three years;

- seizure types that include myoclonic (jerk) or atonic (drop) seizures;

- seizures that are initially difficult to control;

- the need for more than one anti-epileptic drug to obtain control of the seizures;

- the association of other neurological problems, such as moderate or severe learning difficulties, or a physical handicap such as cerebral palsy; and

- if a cause has been identified (e.g. abnormal development of the brain, as in tuberous sclerosis (p. 28), or following meningitis or encephalitis (pp. 36–7).

There are other factors which indicate a good prognosis. These include:

- epilepsy that starts after 5 but before 13 years of age;
- seizure types that include typical absence (petit mal) seizures or tonic–clonic (grand mal) seizures;
- ready control of seizures, using just one anti-epileptic drug;
- a lack of other associated neurological problems;
- the absence of an identified cause; and
- the presence of a strong family history of epilepsy.

Many of the epilepsies in children can be classified into epilepsy syndromes. One of the purposes of this classification is to give some guidance on the prognosis or outcome. Syndromes that have a poor prognosis include the West syndrome (the seizure type in which is infantile spasms or myoclonic seizures) and the Lennox–Gastaut syndrome (seizure types include atonic, tonic, and myoclonic seizures). Seizures in both these syndromes start before the age of 3 years (rarely between 3 and 7 years in Lennox–Gastaut syndrome), and this in itself carries an unfavourable prognosis. Syndromes that have a good outcome include typical absence epilepsy (petit mal) (p. 13) and some partial epilepsies (for example, benign partial epilepsy with centro-temporal (rolandic) spikes). In typical absence epilepsy, between 70 and 75 per cent of children will stop having absence seizures by the age of 14–16 years and the anti-epileptic medication can be withdrawn. The remaining 25–30 per cent may need to continue taking medication into adult life, perhaps even for the rest of their life. The children that are likely to fall into this group are those in whom absences began after the age of 11 or 12 years, were associated with generalized tonic–clonic (grand mal) seizures, and in whom the seizures were difficult to control.

Benign partial epilepsy with centro-temporal (rolandic) spikes is, as the name suggests, really benign. All the children with this epilepsy syndrome will have stopped having seizures by 14–16 years of age, and medication can be withdrawn with no risk of relapse (recurrence) of seizures.

Some syndromes have an intermediate outlook. One of these is juvenile myoclonic epilepsy which usually starts between 10 and 16 years of age. The seizures (myoclonic and generalized tonic–clonic) are usually easily controlled by one drug (sodium valproate), but if the medication is withdrawn, the seizures may recur. Many (but not all) patients who have this type of epilepsy will have to take the treatment for the rest of their lives.

Overall, approximately 30–40 per cent of children will 'outgrow' their epilepsy before they become an adult. This means that the anti-epileptic medication can be withdrawn. Over 70 per cent of children with typical absence epilepsy will probably be able to have their medication withdrawn after they have been seizure-free for between two and three years. In contrast, over 90 per cent of children with Lennox–Gastaut syndrome will probably need to take anti-epileptic drugs for most of their lives.

Associated neurological problems

The presence of learning difficulties or physical disabilities in association with epilepsy usually carries a poor outlook. However, this does not necessarily mean either that the epilepsy has caused the additional problems, or that these problems have been responsible for the poor outcome. What it usually means is that the underlying abnormality of the brain (of whatever cause) has been severe enough to produce both an epilepsy which is difficult to treat *and* other neurological problems.

Long-term outlook in adults

The factors which predict a poor outlook in adults are also well-known. The first is that if the epilepsy is initially difficult to control, then it will usually continue to be difficult to control. The longer that seizures have continued, the less likely they are to stop. Other poor prognostic factors include evidence of structural damage, as manifest by associated neurological signs, the occurrence of partial seizures and the occurrence of episodes of status epilepticus. Exceptions to this general rule are that neurological signs and seizures arising as a result of strokes in older age are not generally difficult to control.

Stopping anti-epileptic medication

Children with epilepsy and their parents, and adults with epilepsy obviously want to know when it is sensible to stop anti-epileptic medication when they have been free of seizures for two or three years. What risks of recurrence do they have, and should they stop the drugs very slowly, or does the speed with which they do this matter very much? As Fig. 7.1 shows, 20 years after diagnosis, 50 per cent of a community sample will have been free from all seizures without anti-epileptic drugs for at least five years, and many will have abandoned their drugs far earlier. What advice can be given?

First of all, it must be recognized that many people are anxious about the possibility of recurrence of seizures, not least because if one occurs, a driving licence regained will be lost again for one year. However, it seems sensible to try and avoid potential adverse effects from very long-term use. In children, there may be anxieties about continued medication and potential effects on cognitive function and learning. Women in their child-bearing years may be anxious about the possible effects of anti-epileptic drugs upon the prenatal development of their babies.

Factors which indicate a significant risk of relapse of seizures on stopping anti-epileptic drugs include the epilepsy syndrome (juvenile myoclonic epilepsy being particularly likely to relapse), and the duration of epilepsy, the number of tonic–clonic seizures so far, and the need to take more than one anti-epileptic drug before control was established. All these factors, if present, suggest 'difficult' epilepsy, so it is not surprising if seizures recur if anti-epileptic drugs are stopped.

The EEG may occasionally be helpful about deciding when to withdraw drugs but only in children, in whom it has been shown that the presence of persisting generalized spike-wave activity makes relapse more likely. The evidence is much less impressive in adults,

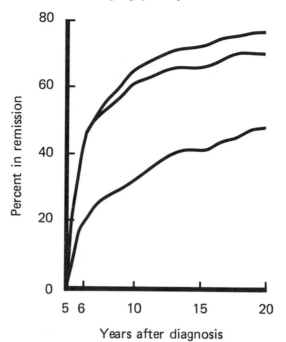

Fig. 7.1 Remission of epilepsy.

Top curve: probability of completing a period of five consecutive years without seizures. For example, six years after diagnosis 42 per cent of patients have been seizure free for five years.

Middle curve: the probability of being in remission, at any time, for at least the past five years. The difference between the top and middle curve is due to relapse after achievement of a five-year remission. For example at 20 years after diagnosis 70 per cent of patients are currently free from seizures and have been for five years and a further 6 per cent have had at least one seizure-free period of at least five years' duration, but have subsequently relapsed.

Lowest curve: the probability of being free of seizures for at least five years whilst not taking anticonvulsant drugs.

In summary, 20 years after diagnosis 50 per cent of patients were free from seizures without anticonvulsants for at least five years. A further 20 per cent continue to take anticonvulsant medication and have also been free of seizures for at least five years. Seizures continue, in spite of medication, in 30 per cent. Data from Dr J.F. Annegers and colleagues.

but it may be assumed that a markedly abnormal EEG, by indicating widespread nerve cell abnormalities, makes it rather more likely that further seizures will occur. However, the finding of any abnormality does not imply that seizures necessarily will recur, and the absence of any abnormality does not guarantee that seizures will not recur. For this reason, many specialists do not carry out an EEG before stopping treatment, but decide on the basis of the type of seizure or epilepsy syndrome that the patient has and the interval that the patient has been seizure-free.

It is generally felt, if a decision is made to withdraw anti-epileptic drugs, this should be done gradually over about two–three months or so. This is particularly important for phenobarbitone and for the benzodiazepine group of drugs (for example, diazepam or Valium and clobazam frizium) of drugs; in patients taking these drugs, abrupt withdrawal may precipitate a burst of seizures, rather like what is known to happen in someone who suddenly stops drinking after many years of abusing alcohol.

8 Living with epilepsy

What to do during a seizure

What should a bystander do during a grand mal attack? The onset is often so sudden that it is difficult to do much at all in the early stage, though it may be possible to break the person's fall. Parents or other relatives may recognize the warning signs that may occur if the generalized seizure follows a focal discharge, and so may have time to help the person to a chair or to a bed before the grand mal begins.

Don't try to open the person's clenched mouth. The tongue, if bitten, is bitten at the onset of the attack, so there is no point in trying to save it. If the bystander uses his own fingers to try to force the mouth open, they may well be bitten in the clonic phase. If he tries to force a spoon or pencil between the teeth, the person's teeth may be damaged. These manoeuvres are still sometimes attempted by tradition, and sometimes, presumably, because it is assumed that the person's blue colour and arrest of breathing are due to obstruction to the passage of air into the lungs. Attempts to 'loosen the collar' presumably result from the same thoughts. However, all of us have enough gaps between our teeth to allow passage of air around them as readers can readily show for themselves by clenching their teeth, pinching the nose, and breathing in. Obstruction to the airway *may* occur during a seizure, if the person is lying on his back. The tongue may then fall backwards into the pharynx, and, for this reason, it is worth turning someone suffering a grand mal seizure into a position halfway between lying on his or her side and face, and thumping the back so that the tongue and any dentures fall forwards. This position also has the advantage that if the person vomits, as occasionally happens, the contents of the stomach pass easily out of the mouth, and there is no danger of vomit entering the trachea and lungs.

If a grand mal seizure occurs in a public place, it usually happens that someone calls an ambulance—very often to the annoyance of the person with epilepsy, who is well on the way to recovery by the time the ambulance driver delivers him to the local hospital. There is no need to call an ambulance unless it is clear that repeated seizures are occurring.

There is usually little to be done during a partial seizure, except to stand by in a reassuring manner until seizure activity ceases. Occasionally gentle restraint may be necessary in the case of complex automatic behaviour (p. 6).

Sensible restrictions on activities

Many relatives of people with epilepsy are naturally concerned as to what may happen during a seizure if they are not present to assist. We have known this anxiety carried to extremes. One of our patients, an epileptic woman of 30, was still sharing her parents' bedroom, as they were concerned that she might come to harm during a nocturnal seizure, even though she had had none for 15 years! In practice, harm resulting from seizures is exceptionally rare, but there are a few sensible precautions.

Children with epilepsy—what can and what can't they do?

We emphasize that the vast majority of children who have epilepsy can take part in all the activities and games that make childhood such fun and an exciting time of life. Unfortunately, many people— including parents, are too afraid and concerned about what may happen *if* a child has an attack, and because of this become over-protective. Being over-protective is, in some ways, more of a danger to the child than not caring enough; children may never learn to do things for themselves, may never be involved in decisions about their own treatment and may never develop the necessary skills to become independent. This is very important because parents will not be around for ever to care for their children.

Swimming is perfectly safe, providing it is not done alone, but with someone who knows what to do if a seizure does occur in the pool; a swimming-pool attendant must also be told. The child should not swim in deep or very cold water, and if in the sea, should be within wading distance of land. For sailing obviously a life-jacket should be worn.

Cycling and horse riding are popular activities, and safety helmets should be worn by everyone who cycles or rides, whether or not they have epilepsy. Care should be taken when cycling on a busy road or in traffic, and ideally horse riders should not ride alone, in case of an accident.

Most children enjoy climbing—whether it is trees, rocks and cliffs on the beach, or apparatus in the gym at school. Where the child's epilepsy is fully controlled, then climbing is usually safe. However, it is probably unwise to climb mountains (using ropes) either alone or with friends, as the risk of severe injuries (to others as well as oneself) is greater if there is a fall due to a seizure.

Sports such as badminton, squash, tennis, hockey, and football are likely to be entirely safe. It is reasonable to take part in contact sports such as rugby and wrestling, but boxing is best avoided. A very small proportion of people with epilepsy may have seizures triggered by flashing or flickering lights, particularly if they are tired. Certain precautions should be taken when playing video games or even when watching television pp. 44–5. These include the following:

- sitting at least three feet (if playing a video game) or ten feet (if watching television) from the screen;

- when changing TV channels use a remote control unit, or if there is no remote control, one eye should be covered as the channel is changed;

- the video game should not be played in a dark room; a bright light should be on in the room; and the video game should not be played for more than an hour at a time, nor late at night when tired.

The use of computers or word processors for work either at home or school only rarely causes seizures and they may be used safely.

Most parents of children who do not have epilepsy will encourage adventures and taking part in activities, whilst taking sensible precautions to reduce the risk of injury, but there are always certain hazards—and accidents do happen, such as falling off bicycles, off playground equipment, or out of trees. It is important that parents do not become too anxious or worried about these risks, just because their child has epilepsy. Some families live in constant fear of the recurrence of a seizure—in the home, at school, or just outside playing. This fear is very easily detected by children, so that everyone becomes afraid of epilepsy and further seizures. Other parents may be ashamed of their child's epilepsy and will never talk about it; this is very unfortunate and will frequently cause the child to become isolated, withdrawn, and ashamed of having epilepsy. This may then limit their expectations and opportunities in life.

Education

Most children with epilepsy attend normal mainstream schools and can participate fully in the schools' curricular and extra-curricular activities. This is the case even in children in whom the epilepsy is not fully controlled. It is important for the teachers and for the school doctor and nurse to know that a child has epilepsy—even if the child's seizures are at the current time controlled. Teachers will then know what to expect and what to do if the child has a seizure. The teacher may also involve children in the class in the care of the child after a seizure; this is important for two reasons. First, it teaches children how to help someone in a seizure, and secondly—and perhaps more importantly—it shows children that there is no need to be scared or upset when someone has a fit. Hopefully, such activities may reduce, in future generations, some of the misunderstanding and social prejudice which surround epilepsy.

About one fifth of children with epilepsy are not able to attend a normal school. This may simply be because of different and frequent seizure types which are not fully controlled. However, the more common reason for these children not being able to attend a normal school is that they have additional problems, such as moderate or severe learning difficulties or physical handicaps (or both), as well as their epilepsy. Most of these children will attend special schools, usually within the local neighbourhood. In this situation in the

UK, under the terms of the Education Act, the child will have an assessment or 'statement' made of his or her educational needs so that the most appropriate school can be found. This statement is based on reports from doctors (including the hospital doctor), teachers, clinical psychologists, therapists, and any other specialist who may have been involved with the child. The ultimate decision as to which school the child should attend rests with the parent.

Perhaps 1–2 per cent of all children with epilepsy may need to attend a school specifically established for children with epilepsy. These schools are usually residential or boarding schools, and the staff have special expertise in teaching children with epilepsy, in coping with their seizures, and in generally supporting them. One of the additional benefits provided by these schools is that they allow separation from the family. The benefit of this lies in the over-protective attitude of many parents who do not allow their child the opportunity to participate in normal social activities. This clearly may not be in the child's best interest with regard to either control of seizures or enabling the child to 'grow' into adulthood and to develop a degree of independence. The environment provided by these schools encourages self-reliance.

Occasionally, a child with epilepsy, although not having frequent seizures, may be doing badly in school. Rarely this is due to the fact that the child is experiencing many more absences or complex partial seizures. These may actually be first picked up by the child's teachers. In these situations, an EEG may help to confirm that the child is experiencing frequent seizures. Another rare possibility—but one that is often put forward—is that the child's poor school work is due to the effect of the anti-epileptic drugs. However, if the child is not excessively sleepy or drowsy, then it is most unlikely that the drugs are interfering significantly with school work. Exceptions include phenobarbitone and phenytoin, which may affect a child's concentration and therefore their learning potential. In these situations the amount of drug in the blood may need to be checked. The most common reason for learning problems in a child with epilepsy is that the intellectual difficulty and the epilepsy share a common cause due to abnormal development of the brain or brain damage (for example, after meningitis or a head injury). In these situations, an educational psychologist will assess the child's strengths and weaknesses and advise on the most appropriate school (this is the statement of a child's educational needs mentioned on p. 118). Sometimes the cause of the child's learning difficulties may be familial—that is, other family members show similar educational problems which has nothing at all to do with the epilepsy.

Children up until the age of 16 years are well cared for by society, educationally and medically. The difficult time comes after the age of 16 years—the 'adolescent' period which, brings changes in social, family, and educational life. This is often a difficult time of life, even for those who do not have epilepsy.

Many changes occur at adolescence which need to be coped with.

- The seizures may change in type, particularly if the epilepsy started at a young age. These changes may include more complex partial and generalized tonic–clonic seizures, and a reduction in absence and myoclonic (jerk) seizures.

- The anti-epileptic medication may have to change in order to maintain control of the epileptic seizures. This may mean a change in dose or even the introduction of different drugs.

- Young people may find it difficult to take their anti-epileptic drug regularly, or they may deliberately decide not to do so. This is more likely to occur in teenagers who have recently been diagnosed and who may find it difficult to come to terms with the diagnosis and need for regular treatment. This may be just one part of a general rebelliousness—against the condition, the treatment, the doctor, family and friends, even life itself. The best way of dealing with these understandable reactions is for the young person to talk about their epilepsy and all its associated problems. Friends may or may not be the easiest to talk to, but hopefully the young person will discuss his or her feelings with the rest of the family and with an understanding doctor.

- There are a number of educational possibilities beyond the normal school leaving age. Many young people with epilepsy will obtain higher qualifications at school and then obtain a place at college or university. It is important that college or university tutors and examiners are told about students who have epilepsy as this promotes and encourages increased awareness and understanding. Those students who live away from home in halls of residence or in rented accommodation should tell friends and college or university tutors.

• Most paediatricians would not think it sensible to continue seeing patients over the age of 16 years. Teenagers of 17 or 18 years have questions and needs that reflect his transition to adult life. All too often transfer from paediatric to adult services in poorly planned. The family doctor will continue his or her support, but consideration of course should be given to transferring care to a neurologist who has a special interest in epilepsy. A special clinic for teenagers with epilepsy has been established in Liverpool to ensure that there is a smooth handover of care from a children's epilepsy clinic to an adult clinic, and in which the specific issues and problems of teenagers can be dealt with satisfactorily.

• There are many changes in life style at adolescence, with different interests and activities and different sleeping patterns, and it is known that deprivation of sleep and alcohol may precipitate seizures. These activities are important in developing independence and self reliance. There are few activities which young people with epilepsy cannot undertake.

An occasional drink containing alcohol is unlikely to be harmful. However, alcohol can make anti-epileptic medication less effective and may, in excess, bring on a seizure. It is important to get the balance right—and this applies to the correct amount of sleep and appropriate diet, as well as the amount of alcohol that is drunk. Medical research suggests that drinking more than two units of alcohol in less than 12–15 hours may significantly increase the risk of seizures in patients who have epilepsy (2 units = one pint of beer, lager, or cider, **or** 2 glasses of wine, **or** two measures ('shorts') of spirits such as whisky, rum, vodka, or gin).

• Contraception will also begin to emerge as an important issue during this time. The most effective form of contraception is the pill. The oral contraceptive pill does not make epileptic seizures more or less likely to happen and there is no reason why women with epilepsy cannot take the pill. However, as has already been discussed on p. 95, certain anti-epileptic drugs (except sodium valproate and the newer ones including vigabatrin and gabapertin) may reduce the contraceptive efficacy of the pill, resulting in an unwanted pregnancy. A contraceptive pill with a high oestrogen content may need to be prescribed, but other forms of contraception (condom or cap plus spermicide) should be considered.

Epilepsy as a social weapon

Families must be aware of ways in which epilepsy can be 'used'. The child or young person with epilepsy, knowing of his parents' anxiety about him, may manipulate them into granting him unreasonable requests. They may give in to feeling sorry for his difficulties, or they may feel that they should avoid an emotional upset that might precipitate a seizure. There is no reason why a child with epilepsy should not experience the same discipline as his siblings, who will themselves become jealous and unruly if they feel that one member of the family is being spoiled.

The other side of the coin is that parents may use the threat of epilepsy as a means of controlling behaviour which they otherwise cannot control. Examples we have met include limiting the hours of television watched, and the lateness of the hour by which an adolescent with epilepsy must return home.

Prejudice, and telling others about epilepsy

It is unfortunately true that those with epilepsy do encounter a fair amount of prejudice against them, especially in the field of employment (p. 126). This prejudice is perhaps based on dimly held knowledge of those in special care, or institutions, with the very worst epilepsy, often in association with mental retardation due to major neurological disease.

Prejudice against those with other illnesses is rare. No one minds if you have only one kidney or varicose veins. Most people go out of their way to help a blind person, or someone in a wheelchair. However, a blind or physically disabled person is immediately perceived as 'different'. Bystanders can make judgements about his abilities. They may relate to him in a special way—a manner which is instantly perceived and resented by an occupant of the wheelchair! Such a visible handicap is perceived and managed as such by society. Someone with epilepsy, however, is perfectly normal for 99.9 per cent of the time. His 'handicap' is invisible. He then discredits himself, as it were, by having a seizure. His acquaintances feel deceived. The man they thought was a bank manager turns out to be 'really an epileptic', passing himself off as normal. Such an attitude is ridiculous, yet there is persistent evidence for it. Such prejudice will, we hope, gradually fade, as misconceptions about epilepsy are dispelled. However, it would be foolish to deny its existence at the present time.

A major problem that someone with epilepsy has to decide, therefore, is how much to tell, and to whom. For example, no mother wants to tell everyone that her son has epilepsy, but if the boy is staying the night at the house of a friend, it is only sensible to let his friend's parents know that he might have a seizure, and to tell them how to cope. Most parents would agree with this policy if the boy was having seizures every fortnight or so—but what if they occurred only every six months? Parents might feel that they were spoiling the boy's chances of friendship and social development if they sent him off with the label of epilepsy around his neck.

Young people with epilepsy forming friendships with the opposite sex also suffer agonies about these decisions. If the epilepsy is not talked about early in the relationship the subject becomes more and more difficult to bring up. The problem may then be revealed by the occurrence of a seizure without prior explanation. Both parties feel devastated—the one guilty and ashamed at not having had the courage to explain the problem, the other surprised and ashamed of their surprise and inability to cope both with the seizure and their own feelings about it.

On balance, we are sure that it is best for a person with epilepsy to tell those he meets frequently something of the facts, so that they can cope if a seizure occurs. Friends will appreciate the confidence shown in them by the fact of this disclosure.

Psychological disorders and epilepsy

People with epilepsy have to cope with the effects of their seizures on their chances in life—which may well be reduced if seizures are frequent. Throughout all of life with epilepsy, they have to act as their own public relations officer, deciding how much to tell and how much to conceal. Their circle of friends and choice of sexual partner may well be narrowed. Their inability to hold a driving licence and limitations in employment reduce their earning power, social status, and long-term financial security. By avoidance of factors which they believe may precipitate seizures, social activities may be greatly reduced. It is not surprising, therefore, that people with epilepsy become anxious, or depressed, or resentful and irritable.

The age of onset of epilepsy influences the psychological effects suffered. A robust man of 45 in previous good health who develops epilepsy following a head injury has established his personality, social life, family, and employment before the injury. Although he may encounter problems with future employment, there is no change in how his friends and family perceive him and react to him. The late age of onset and the clear-cut cause of seizures allows this man and his family to take up the position that although he may have a few blackouts he is not really 'an epileptic'.

It is quite different for a girl whose epilepsy begins at the age of 12, with frequent seizures throughout her school career. Whatever her abilities, her friends and teachers perceive her as 'an epileptic'. Epilepsy dominates social intercourse, the development of personality, and possibilities of future employment and establishment of married life. Such a person will have more profound psychological difficulties than the 45-year-old man described above. Anxiety, depression, and resentment are entirely comprehensible reactions to the fact of epilepsy. One might say: 'I would feel like that if I had her problems'. To that extent, therefore, it would be wrong to categorize these psychological effects as an illness, though that does not mean that advice and support from friends, or the family doctor, or a psychiatrist may not aid the person with epilepsy to come to terms with their disability. However skilled the counsellor, we are convinced that the ability to cope depends primarily upon the strength of personality of the person with epilepsy.

Occasionally depression in association with epilepsy may become so severe that treatment with an antidepressant drug is indicated. For reasons discussed on p. 43, this drug should be chosen with care.

Depression and inability to cope with the life situation caused by epilepsy may be so severe as to cause the unfortunate sufferer to take his own life. Suicide is approximately five times more common in those with epilepsy than in the general population.

A psychotic illness with symptoms similar to those of paranoid schizophrenia may occasionally be seen in those with epilepsy arising from a temporal lobe lesion. The occurrence of the psychosis is not necessarily related to the frequency of seizures. Indeed, there is a curious group of patients in whom the psychosis becomes prominent as seizures settle, only to remit as seizures return.

One cause of epilepsy is impaired fetal development of the brain or brain damage occurring at or around the time of birth (pp. 31–2). Children with such brain damage may be less intelligent than their siblings, be more easily distracted from work and play, and be prone to emotional extremes. Because of constant restlessness, this behaviour is sometimes known as the 'hyperkinetic (or hyperactive) syndrome'. It should be understood that both the behaviour and the epilepsy share a common cause; the epilepsy in itself does *not* cause this behaviour.

Problems for women with epilepsy

Problems facing women with epilepsy have been referred to at various places within the book. The effect of menstruation on seizure frequency is discussed on p. 42. The interaction between anticonvulsant drugs and oral contraceptives is discussed on p. 95. The effects of anticonvulsant drugs on the fetus are discussed on pp. 92–3.

Some mothers report that their seizures become more frequent, others less frequent during pregnancy, and others have seizures which remain more or less unchanged in pregnancy. There seems no way of predicting what is going to happen in the first pregnancy, except that those with very frequent seizures are, unfortunately, likely to get worse. By and large, subsequent pregnancies in any one mother follow much the same pattern. An unexpected and totally unexplained finding has been that those pregnant with a male baby are rather more likely to have more frequent seizures. Although epilepsy may start for the first time during pregnancy, this usually seems to be coincidental, and there is no good evidence that pregnancy itself is a particularly potent event in *inducing* seizures. One possible reason for an increase in frequency of seizures during pregnancy is that the body processes anticonvulsant drugs differently. The interactions between pregnancy and drug metabolism may be complex.

Some anti-epileptic drugs pass through the placenta into the fetus. Phenobarbitone is perhaps the best-known example. After delivery the baby's serum phenobarbitone falls, and during the early days after birth the baby may be much more fractious and irritable than most new-born babies.

Many mothers on anti-epileptic drugs wonder whether they can breast-feed their babies. Careful studies have been made on this point, and only small quantities of the drugs are secreted into milk, so it is quite safe to breast-feed.

Sexual activity and epilepsy

Orgasm in both men and women is presumably accompanied by some sort of 'paroxysmal discharge of cerebral nerve cells'. This, and the impossibility of control of orgasm beyond a certain point, suggests an analogy with seizures. In fact seizures during or immediately after intercourse are exceptionally uncommon. When they do occur, they probably represent one of the types of reflex epilepsy described on p. 44. Except in these rarer cases, there is certainly no reason for avoiding intercourse on the grounds that seizures may be provoked.

Unfortunately, epilepsy is sometimes accompanied by a decline in sexuality. Many adolescents find their initial dates worrying enough ('Which cinema should I take her to?' 'Should I let him kiss me?'), but how much more worrying must it be to take a girl out knowing that there is a chance, albeit a remote chance, that a seizure will occur during the date? Anxiety about contact with the opposite sex may have its basis in such entirely understandable problems of adolescence. However, there is evidence that a decline in sexuality may occur more frequently in those with seizures arising in the temporal lobe than in other types of seizures. Rarely, libido and potency may improve after temporal lobe surgery.

Sometimes patients may complain about loss of libido and sexual performance after beginning anticonvulsant drugs. This seems to happen most frequently after phenobarbitone and primidone, but it is difficult to be sure how much is due to the drugs, and how much to social and psychological factors.

Employment

It is not sensible to be a steeple-jack or scaffolder if one has many seizures. But just what restrictions on employment should be applied to those with epilepsy?

First of all, there are the legal restrictions on driving, which are fully discussed on p. 131. This may stop employment as a travelling representative, for example, but these Regulations have a wider effect in making travel to a job more difficult, especially in rural areas, however suitable that job may be.

Driving is the most obvious way in which a person with epilepsy can harm others, as well as himself, during a seizure. But there are occupations of heavy personal responsibility to others which those with uncontrolled seizures must not do. Surgery and nursing are obvious examples from our own health professions. The occupations of airline pilot, and bus, train, mass transit and crane driver, railway signalman, and merchant navy sailor, are other examples. The Armed Forces, fire, and ambulance services and Police also exclude those with continuing seizures.

In other jobs, there is no real risk to bystanders during a seizure, but there is a substantial risk of injury or death to the person with continuing epilepsy. The operation of heavy moving machinery, including agricultural machinery, work near conveyor belts, work at heights, particularly in the construction or electric power industries, and work underground or underwater should all be avoided. However keen the subject may be to take his own life in his hands, it is not fair to burden employers if there is a substantial risk of a mutilating or fatal accident.

One of the agonizing questions that people with infrequent seizures must ask themselves is whether to tell a potential employer about them. Obviously it is best if they do because the employer can take into account any remote risks about which the applicant is unaware. Employers can make an occasional allowance for rare but unexpected absences from work, and they can, in an informed way, cope with occasional seizures at work. The truth of the matter is that many employers reject those with seizures which are few and far between, or those who have had no seizures for some years, for jobs which carry virtually no risk to the person with epilepsy or to others.

Surveys of public attitudes towards those with epilepsy are in our view meaningless, insofar as potential employers may well make favourable remarks about the employment of a hypothetical person with epilepsy in response to an interviewer, because this is the polite and modern thing to say. However, it is their actual behaviour in hiring and firing that counts. A truer measure of the amount of prejudice against employing people with epilepsy would be to send round two personable young people with equal qualifications in response to 100 advertisements for a post as a secretary, for example. In half the interviews each applicant would indicate that they suffered from mild, well-controlled epilepsy. The success rate with and without revealing this information would be a fair guide to current prejudice against the employment of those with epilepsy. Unfortunately such a study would be unethical, insofar as it would waste the time and resources of employers. Nevertheless, we would be fascinated to know the answer!

Those with epilepsy intuitively know the likely result from the results of their own interviews. One survey of people with epilepsy in London showed that over half those who had two or more full-time jobs after the onset of epilepsy had never disclosed their epilepsy to an employer, and only one in ten had *always* revealed it. Furthermore, if seizures were infrequent or nocturnal, so that applicants considered that they had a good chance of getting away with concealment, the employer was virtually never informed. Whilst not condoning or encouraging dishonesty, the relative success of this policy can be judged by the fact that 74 per cent of the men of employable age with epilepsy were employed at the time of the survey, compared with 81 per cent of male workers of the same age group in the UK as a whole.

Whatever the policy about disclosure, applicants for a job will be more successful if they follow the general rules of taking care with their written application, taking trouble to inform themselves about the responsibilities of the post and about the employer, presenting themselves well at interviews, selling their ability to do the job, and convincing the prospective employer that they have an enthusiastic desire to work. What is absolutely disastrous is for frequent rejections to lead to the development of a chip on the shoulder, so that a potential employer is confronted by the attitude 'I have epilepsy; you haven't; you have a duty to employ me'. We have helped look after patients with seizures who succeed in presenting themselves and their epilepsy in such an unfavourable light that we feel there can be no strong motivation to obtain work.

Obtaining a job is obviously only the first step. Most of us want promotion up to the limits of our energies and capabilities, and here again epilepsy, even if well controlled, often spoils chances in life. It is difficult to measure the frequency with which those well qualified for promotion are overlooked, but one study found that the rate of dismissal following the onset of epilepsy was increased approximately sixfold.

There is another more subtle way in which epilepsy can hinder employment and promotion. The fear of encountering rejection, or the fear of leaving an established position with a tolerant employer may cause the people with epilepsy to deny themselves chances for betterment. Just as the employer may be prejudiced against 'epileptics' so may the epileptic be prejudiced against 'employers', believing them all to be lacking in understanding.

There may be an advantage in young people with epilepsy seeking a career in small organizations, where regulations for employment, sick leave, insurance, and pensions are flexible compared with those of, for example, the Civil Service.

As might be expected, if seizures occur frequently, one study showed that it was much more difficult to hold down a job. The study showed that a third of the unemployed were having generalized seizures monthly or more frequently, whilst only 2 per cent of those in work were suffering equivalently. Roughly the same proportions held true for partial seizures. Apart from seizure frequency, the main barrier to employment is lack of any special skill. One survey found, as could have been foretold, that virtually all those with frequent seizures and no special skills were unemployed. It is here that specialist advice from employment agencies should be sought.

In the UK the Employment Service provides a wide range of services to help people with disabilities to get and keep suitable employment. Most disabled people helped by the Employment Service are helped by general services. There is also a network of 71 Placing, Assessment, and Counselling Teams (PACTs) to help those people with disabilities who cannot be helped properly by the general services. This may include some people with epilepsy. People in PACTs are called Disability Employment Advisers (DEAs). The DEA can be contacted at, or through, the local Employment Service Jobcentre. It is not necessary to be registered as disabled to use most of the services provided through the DEA, though they may recommend registration. The Disabled Persons Register is a voluntary register of people who want to work, and are able to do so, but who have difficulty in getting or keeping suitable work because of their long-term health problem or disability. The Register is run by the Employment Service through its DEAs. All employers who have 20 or more workers have a duty, under the Disabled Persons (Employment) Acts 1944 and 1958, to employ a quota of registered disabled people, usually three per cent of their total workforce. Consequently a big firm is keen to employ someone capable of good work if they happen to be on the Register. Before registration, the family doctor or neurologist will, with the person's consent, fill in a special form which provides basic information about the type and frequency of seizures, and any other associated disability.

The DEA may consider that a person with epilepsy may benefit from a course of vocational training, to equip him or her with a special skill not already possessed. For example, a nurse with frequent seizures might no longer be suitable for nursing, until the seizures were controlled, and the DEA might well advise that she or he take a course to encourage the development of business skills. This could be arranged through, and at the expense of, the local Training and Enterprise Council (TEC) (Local Enterprise Company (LEC) in Scotland). Training allowances may be payable. The DEA could put the client in touch with the TEC (LEC).

For those with frequent seizures, possibly in association with learning disabilities, the DEA may advise a job in Supported Employment, in which severely handicapped people work in a supported environment—either in a Remploy factory, a supported workshop run by a local authority or voluntary body, or in a supported placement in ordinary employment.

The DEA can also advise on the wide range of help which is available, where appropriate, through the new Access to Work Programme. Individuals can get up to £21 000 worth of help, over a five year period, to pay for things such as extra costs of travel to work for those who cannot use public transport because of their disability; vehicle adaptations; special equipment needed at work; adaptations to the employer's premises; communication support for blind or deaf people at work; or human support. The DEA can also offer a weekly grant to an employer who provides employment on a trial basis to give a disabled person the chance to demonstrate that they can do the job.

There will always be a nucleus of people with epilepsy who are unemployed either temporarily or more or less permanently. The person who is capable of work but unemployed may, as time passes, become progressively more unemployable if not given occupation and support. It is here that local authority social workers DEAs, and epilepsy associations can help.

Driving and epilepsy

There are few aspects of having epilepsy in adult life that cause greater distress than the necessary legal restrictions on driving. For some people owning and using a car is a hobby in itself—albeit an expensive one. Others, particularly those living in rural areas where public transport is limited or non-existent, find car ownership and driving necessary for shopping and social contact, and for getting to work. There are jobs such as delivery van driver in which driving is the sole function of employment, and any restriction on driving will cause the employee to lose his job.

This book may well be read in a number of countries, and the legal requirements vary from place to place. As an example, however, we consider the UK eligibility to hold a private (Group 1) driving licence in the UK , as determined by the Motor Vehicles (Driving Licences) (Amendment) (No. 2) Regulations 1994 which came into force on 5th August 1994. Epilepsy is prescribed for the purposes of Sections [92 (4) (b)] of the 1988 Road Traffic Act. The 1994 Regulations amended the 1987 Regulations (which specified a seizure-free period of two years) as follows:

'An applicant for a licence suffering from epilepsy shall satisfy the following conditions, namely that he shall—

a) have been free from any epileptic attack during the period of one year immediately preceding the date when the licence is granted; or

b) have had an epileptic attack whilst asleep more than three years before the date when the licence is granted and shall have had attacks only whilst asleep between the date of that attack and the date when the licence is granted;

and that the driving of a vehicle by him in accordance with the licence is not likely to be a danger to the public.'

The purpose of clause (b) is to allow someone to drive who has established a long history of seizures whilst asleep without ever having had any whilst awake. It allows someone with continuing seizures only whilst asleep to drive, without requiring a period of one year free from such a seizure.

These Regulations are, we believe, a reasonable attempt to protect the public from the chances of meeting a driver who is briefly incapable of controlling his car because of a seizure. The Regulations are also fair to those with epilepsy insofar as they clearly state the circumstances under which they can drive.

What actually happens in practice? Take the example of a woman who has held a licence for several years, and then has two grand mal seizures at work within a month. Her family doctor or neurologist will explain that she is no longer eligible to hold a driving licence. It is not the responsibility of either doctor to inform the licensing authority of this, but a doctor will record in their notes the fact that they have explained the position to the patient. It is the driver's responsibility to take action. Inside each UK Driving Licence is the statement that the 'Drivers Medical Branch, Swansea SA99 1TU MUST be told at once if: you NOW have any physical or mental disability which affects your fitness as a driver or which might do so IN THE FUTURE'. The patient should write a brief note to the Drivers and Vehicle Licensing Authority (DVLA) at Swansea (the address above being sufficient) explaining the details and enclosing the licence, which will be acknowledged. No further action is necessary.

If all goes well for this woman, and she has no further seizures after the first two, she becomes eligible to hold a driving licence one year after the date of the last attack. She then completes an application form as usual. In Section 6d, or in a covering letter if there is insufficient space on the form, she writes briefly exactly what has occurred, refers to her earlier letter, states the date of her last seizure, and gives the name and address of her family doctor or neurologist to whom reference can be made. After a short interval, she will receive her new licence.

All this seems entirely straightforward, but we know that many people with epilepsy find the Regulations hard to accept. Doctors appreciate the difficulties that may be caused by giving up driving. Driving is usually an essential part of their work, so they do not have to make great leaps of imagination to realize the difficulties that a ban on driving may cause. Unfortunately the law does not take hardship into account. Doctors should, however, not only advise their patients of the law, but also, from their experience, advise patients how to cope with their changed circumstances. Doctors are in a position to influence decisions of employers about the nature of their patients' work. They can write to the employer, with the patient's consent, supporting a request for a change of job within the same company. In such a letter, a doctor does not necessarily have to say that the person has epilepsy, only that they are not able to drive for medical reasons, and not likely to be able to drive for some time. Such letters may well influence company decisions. We have known many examples of this. A travelling salesman has become a successful office-bound sales manager; a busy surveyor has taken on increased training responsibilities; and a delivery van driver has been employed within the factory making the goods he was previously delivering. Obviously such changes are easier within large organizations with their greater variety of jobs.

We usually advise people living in rural areas not to move house just because of their new inability to drive. If it seems likely that the seizures can be easily controlled, then it is probably better to cope somehow for the time necessary, rather than disturb the whole family's way of life. The people with epilepsy are the only ones who can decide whether to move, but their doctors should give them sufficient information about the probability of seizure control to allow an informed decision.

Sometimes people with epilepsy will say that they consider it safe to drive as they always get a warning of their attacks. Leaving aside the legal point—that they are ineligible, and unfortunately their opinion does not count—we explain that the warning is the start of the cerebral events which form the early part of the seizure itself. The fact that to date the progression of the seizure discharge has been sufficiently slow to allow the subject to stop his or her car safely does not mean that this will always be the case. Such a person with epilepsy may well have a sudden grand mal seizure without warning.

Again, people with epilepsy may indicate that they consider it safe to drive, as all their seizures are small ones—perhaps temporal lobe seizures in which consciousness is disturbed in only a minor way. We have to say that the law does not distinguish between the various types of seizures. We also have to say that the next seizure may unfortunately be a grand mal one, and that in any event catastrophe is as likely to be caused by a momentary reduction of conscious awareness as by a major fit.

With the exception of seizures which have always occurred during sleep, about which the Regulations are cited on p. 131, the time of seizure is irrelevant. It is useless for the patient to say to his or her doctor that seizures always occur in the evening, or sometimes even: 'I've never had one whilst driving', as the next seizure may well be when he or she is in the driving seat.

Sometimes a patient may feel that the events which have led him to the doctor are not epileptic in nature. All a doctor can do in such circumstances is to disagree, and advise that the patient seeks a further opinion. As noted above, it is not a doctor's responsibility to inform the licensing authority of a person's epilepsy. It may be, however, that if a doctor is convinced of the diagnosis, and believes that there is a real risk to the public, and if the patient refuses to seek a further opinion, he or she may feel that responsibility to the public at large overrides responsibility to the individual patient.

There are, however, circumstances in which the occurrence of epileptic seizures is not automatically associated with loss of eligibility to hold a driving licence. Clause (b) of the Regulations quoted on p. 131 states that an applicant shall 'have had an epileptic attack whilst asleep more than three years before the date when the licence is granted and shall have had attacks only whilst asleep between the date of that attack and the date when the licence is granted'. There are some people, though not many, who only have fits during sleep; three years seems a reasonable period to allow one to see if that is the case. After that, even if attacks do occur in sleep and never whilst awake, a person can nevertheless drive.

The Regulations are careful to state 'attacks whilst asleep' rather than nocturnal attacks, to take account of those who are on night shift and sleep during the day. The concession to those who have only had attacks whilst asleep is in fact a generous one, insofar as a follow-up study by one neurologist of those who had only had nocturnal seizures showed that about one third had a seizure whilst awake within the next five years. Of course a single seizure of any type whilst awake immediately renders the person who until then has only had seizures whilst asleep ineligible to drive. Likewise a single seizure whilst awake earlier in life prevents the application of this concession even if all subsequent seizures are whilst asleep.

The Regulations state nothing about anti-epileptic medication. The law is, as it were, interested in seizures and not in drugs. This means that there is no need to withdraw medication after a seizure-free interval so that the patient can resume driving. On common-sense grounds it is probably marginally safer to be a passenger with someone who has had seizures in the past, who remains on anti-epileptic medication, rather than travel with someone who had his last seizure three years ago and stopped his drugs yesterday.

The whole area is fraught with difficulties. For example, young adults who have successfully come through a few petit mal and grand mal attacks in childhood may have a few morning myoclonic jerks on rare occasions. Such patients often tell us that there is no detectable disturbances of their consciousness during such jerks. Many patients certainly do not regard such occasional jerks as fits, and yet, as they are the product of a paroxysmal discharge of brain cells, they are, technically, seizures. It is to help in advising on such borderline cases as this that the Department of Transport has available an Honorary Medical Advisory Panel on Epilepsy. It is open to any applicant for a licence who disagrees with the Department's refusal to grant him a licence, on the grounds that he has epilepsy and does not satisfy the requirements of the Regulations, to appeal to the Advisory Panel. From a compilation of the advice given by members of the Panel, a set of guidelines has been drawn up by the Medical Officers of the Department of Transport. If there is doubt in their minds, the matter is referred to the appropriate specialist, and we know that that happens several times each week.

The graph shown on p. 112 indicates that even if a remission of seizures lasting five years has occurred, relapses do unfortunately occur. The relapse rate in the first five years after achieving a remission of five years was 8 per cent. A study organized by the Medical Research Council in the UK has found that about a third of those who stop treatment on medical advice will have a further attack at some time, and of those about a half will have the recurrence within a year. Many will therefore consider it an additional safeguard to continue anti-epileptic medication, if driving, even if they are free from attacks. However, in the same study a number of people had attacks even though they were continuing anti-epileptic drugs so that they could be compared with those who stopped them.

It should also be noted that the 1988 Road Traffic Act prescribes as a relevant disability a liability (*sic*) to seizures. It follows therefore that on occasion a patient who has never had a fit may be ineligible to hold a licence because he is considered liable to have a seizure. A patient with a frontal tumour, or one who has had an intracranial operation, may fall into this category.

Regulations on those who wish to drive heavy good vehicles are even more strict. The current regulations state all of the following criteria must be met. The person must have been free from epileptic attacks for 10 years, have not taken ati-epileptic medication during this 10-year period, and does not have a continuing liability to an epileptic seizure.

Finally, before leaving this vexed question of driving, we should add two further points. So far we have written exclusively about the practice in the UK. The requirements for eligibility vary from country to country, and, in the USA, from state to state. Enquiry must be made of the licensing authority in each country or state in which patients wish to drive. Secondly, we are fully aware that many patients who are ineligible to drive do in fact do so. In one survey of people with epilepsy in Greater London, 12 out of 62 currently ineligible to drive were in fact doing so. This is not always wilful recklessness. Only 3 of the 12 both were aware of the diagnosis, and admitted that they had been told not to drive. Some of the remainder did not realize, so they said, that they had epilepsy, or they felt that they had received explicit or implicit consent to drive from their doctors.

Those who knowingly drive when ineligible must realize that their insurance policies would almost certainly be void if they had an accident. But the terrible risk of killing or maiming another road user or pedestrian should be sufficient discouragement.

There are no restrictions—other than those of common-sense—on riding a pedal bicycle. Even if a rider has a seizure, they are likely to damage only themselves.

Life insurance

One of the few ways that an average person has of building capital throughout his lifetime is by house purchase, by payments into regular saving schemes such as with profits insurance policies and personal equity plans (PEPs) and often by a combination of all these. Couples will also usually wish to provide some sort of monetary support to their surviving partner or children in the event of unexpected early death. In short, life insurance is now regarded as part of nearly everyone's every-day financial arrangements.

Life insurance companies are in business, in the final analysis, to provide a financial return for their shareholders, or, in the case of a Mutual Office, to provide a fair deal for all policy-holders. It has to be admitted that the mortality of *all* those with seizures from *all* causes is higher than the general population. It is therefore not surprising that the Life Offices, if they accept the risk of underwriting the lives of those with epilepsy, require an excess premium to compensate them for the excess risk.

How is this excess premium calculated? The insurance industry uses statistics based on their past experience. As in employment (see p. 128), it is probable that those with a few seizures calculate the risk of 'getting away with' concealment. In a financial transaction such as insurance, concealment of epilepsy is clearly fraudulent, and any policy arranged in this way is void. Insofar as the statistical data of the Life Offices cannot reflect those with a few seizures who have concealed their epilepsy, it is probable that their experience of the mortality of those with declared epilepsy is worse than the true mortality. This experience tends to inflate the excess premium, but we believe that there are other factors. The Offices may be corporately possessed of some of the misconceptions about epilepsy that this book is trying to dispel. Although they employ a medical officer, few if any of these advisers are neurologists, and a single physician can hardly be expected to provide informed and modern statistics about the disease suffered by each and every proposer. Furthermore, the industry as a whole does not distinguish between different types of seizure occurring with different frequencies and due to different causes. In these circumstances the Offices adopt an attitude of 'better be safe than sorry' and charge a premium that is in excess of standard rates.

There is often a considerable difference between the excess rates quoted by various Offices, so it is well worth while seeking professional advice from an insurance broker. For people in the

UK, the firm of Tyser and Company, 12 Camomile Street, London
EC3A 7PT have built up a considerable experience of arranging life
insurance for those with epilepsy. In general, they expect that any
proposer with epilepsy should have been adequately investigated to
exclude a progressive organic cause, and that the proposer should be
reliable at taking his prescribed medication and in following medical
advice. It is very much easier to arrange insurance for those capable
of employment and without intellectual impairment, although in
other cases a quotation can usually be obtained.

We asked Tyser and Company for their views about three specific
examples. Although useful as a general guide, readers must understand that rates will vary as each person with epilepsy is different
both in his problems and in his or her requirements for insurance.

Proposal 1 A man aged 27 next birthday who had frequent seizures in
childhood, several seizures in adolescence, and none over the
last eight years.

Ordinary rates of premium would be allowed for this case, for
any class of Assurance.

Proposal 2 A man aged 33 next birthday who had a single seizure one
year ago. No evidence of any progressive organic disease.

For Term Assurance, where the ordinary rate of premium is
very low, a loading of 50 per cent would be considered by
some Offices. For other types of insurance the market would
consider that a small loading for a short period of one or two
years was justifiable. It might be possible to gain acceptance at
normal rates, and this would be easier if the interval between
the seizures and the proposal were longer.

Proposal 3 A man aged 25 next birthday who has had frequent grand mal
fits since the age of 16, with four fits in the last year.

Assurable, but subject to an extra premium. The actual amount
would probably vary among those Life Offices which are
prepared to accept proposals from those with epilepsy, but
in terms of additional mortality, one underwriter considers
that plus 100 per cent would be a reasonable loading. At
first sight this appears high, but regard should be given to
the very low mortality rate of assured lives at this young age.
In monetary terms the additional premium for Whole of Life
Assurance would be £2.50 per annum for each £1000 of sum

assured. One underwriter's practice would be to limit the term of payment of this extra premium to a period of ten years, but this is by no means general within the industry.

Special care for those with the worst epilepsy

Most people with frequent seizures are looked after at home by devoted parents or partners. Sometimes a fragile situation breaks down and it is clear that a person with epilepsy cannot cope at home. Obviously if it is believed that this is a purely temporary setback likely to be improved by modification of anti-epileptic medication, then the family doctor will arrange a short stay in a neurological unit or in a special centre for epilepsy. Occasionally, however, it is obvious that neither the domestic situation of the person with epilepsy, nor their epilepsy, is going to improve in the foreseeable future, and long-stay care has to be arranged. The precipitating factor is very often the illness or death of the last surviving supporting relative.

In the middle of the last century, an increasing social commitment to those less fortunate than the majority resulted in the establishment of 'colonies' for people with epilepsy. The general plan of such colonies in Europe was of a totally self-contained institution. During the day, the people with epilepsy would work in the open air, in arable and stock farming, and at night they would return to dormitories, or, in the more advanced colonies, to small houses in which some semblance of a family circle was maintained. Many people with severe epilepsy spent the greater part of their lives in such institutions. Unfortunately there is still a need for such long-term care. In the UK there are approximately 2000 people with epilepsy in the former colonies, now called centres for epilepsy, and perhaps another 3000 in other types of residential accommodation supported by local authorities.

An intriguing fact is that about one sixth of those in the epilepsy centres have rare seizures—less often than once a year. Some of these epilepsies have, as it were, burnt themselves out, but the subject has been so long in the institution that they have no base or family circle to which they may return, and the centre is a much-loved home. The other explanation is that epilepsy, although a 'required' disorder for admission to the centres for epilepsy, may not be in itself a great problem—the major reasons for admission being associated impairment of intellect or major physical disability due to brain damage, of which epilepsy is only one symptom. By and large, those in special centres for epilepsy have what has been termed 'epilepsy plus'—epilepsy plus some other major handicap.

The role of the former colonies has gradually changed over the years. First, the word colony, with its implications of dependency, has been dropped, and the name 'centre for epilepsy' has been adopted. Secondly, the centres have established much closer links with university departments of neurological sciences. Indeed much of the best research work in epilepsy in Europe emanates from the former colonies. Thirdly, the centres have taken a greater role in the assessment of patients with severe epilepsy, admitting them for neurological and occupational evaluation for a short period of a few weeks. Fourthly, they are more outward-looking in the employment of people with epilepsy. Sometimes the centre is used as a hostel to which people with epilepsy who can almost, but not quite, manage on their own can return at night.

All this activity does mean that the primary role for which the colonies were established—a sheltered residential home for those people with epilepsy unable to cope outside—is in danger of being submerged. We can tell when this is happening to a centre, because my letter requesting admission for a patient received a reply that the patient 'would not benefit' from residence in the centre. In a small proportion of cases, one has to accept that benefit is not likely to occur, and all that is wanted is a clean, quiet, and kind place to live.

9 *Convulsions associated with fever*

A convulsion which occurs in association with any illness, usually an infection, which causes a rise in temperature (fever) is known as a febrile convulsion.

Febrile convulsions are not a type of epilepsy. In the past it was thought that febrile convulsions could lead to epilepsy but this is now generally believed only rarely to be the case. There are at least three subgroups of febrile convulsions:

(a) The first and largest subgroup is made up of children who have seizures in response to fever as a result of an individual susceptibility that is usually inherited. These children develop normally and have normal EEGs and normal brain scans. This is the group which constitutes 'true' febrile convulsions and will be discussed in detail in this chapter.

(b) The second subgroup comprises children in whom the fever or high temperature acts as a trigger that unmasks epilepsy. In these children, seizures or fits *without* a fever soon develop and the children then can be seen to have definite epilepsy. Magnetic resonance imaging (p. 74) in these children usually shows subtle structural abnormalities, often in one temporal lobe (p. 75). Before their first febrile convulsion, these children may have been developing more slowly than most children.

(c) A very small subgroup comprising children who convulse with fever due to meningitis or encephalitis—meaning respectively an inflammation or infection of the membranes covering the brain, or of the brain substance itself. Obviously it is critically important to recognize this subgroup in order that energetic curative treatment can be started as soon as possible.

'True' febrile convulsions, as defined in (a) above are common: 2–4 per cent of children between the ages of 6 months and 5 years will have at least one febrile convulsion. The most common age is between 12 and 20 months. One should be careful about accepting a diagnosis of a 'true' febrile convulsion in a child aged less than 6 months or older than 5 years—they are more likely to have epilepsy triggered by fever. Girls are more likely than boys to have a febrile convulsion. Up to a third of children who have had one, will have a second febrile convulsion before the age of 5 years.

Most of the convulsions are tonic–clonic (grand mal) in type (see p. 12), and last less than 4–5 minutes. This type of febrile convulsion is called 'simple'. 'Complex' or complicated febrile convulsions are ones that involve only one side of the body, last longer than 15 minutes, or are followed by weakness or loss of use of one side of the body. These 'complex' febrile convulsions are uncommon and account for no more than 10–20 per cent of all 'true' febrile convulsions. Complex febrile convulsions are more commonly seen in children in the other two groups—(b) and (c) described above.

Causes of febrile convulsions

The cause of a febrile convulsion, is, as the name implies, a fever or high temperature. Any of the common childhood infections such as chickenpox, tonsillitis, upper respiratory, ear, bowel or urinary infections may cause a high temperature and therefore cause a febrile convulsion. It is unclear whether it is how quickly the temperature rises, or how high it eventually gets which determines whether a convulsion will occur. Lots of children between 6 months and 5 years of age have febrile illnesses but obviously the majority will not have a convulsion. One of the reasons why some children do, and others do not have convulsions with fever, is because of inherited factors which are important in determining whether febrile convulsions will occur. Almost one third of children will be found to have a family history of febrile convulsions in their parents or siblings (brothers and sisters). When one parent has a history of febrile convulsions, the risk to a child of developing a febrile convulsion is almost 20 per cent; if both parents have a history, then the risk is increased to 50 per cent. The brothers and sisters of a child who has had a febrile convulsion have a three times increased risk of having a febrile convulsion themselves; this risk is even higher in identical twins.

Most children who have febrile convulsions do not need any tests. Usually the cause of the infection and of the fever is obvious from the examination carried out by the doctor—for example, a sore throat (tonsillitis), red ear (otitis media), rash (for example, chickenpox), or cold and cough. Rarely, however, and particularly in children under 18 months of age, a convulsion may be the first sign of meningitis or encephalitis (group (c) above). If there is any doubt as to whether a child has meningitis (particularly in children aged 6–18 months), then a lumbar puncture must be done, and other tests may well be required. Children with simple febrile convulsions do *not* need to have an EEG or brain scan. However, children with complex febrile convulsions (group(b)) may well need them in order to explore what is the underlying cause of their asymmetrical or prolonged convulsion, or earlier slow development.

Treatment

The aims of treatment of febrile convulsion are three-fold:
- to stop the convulsion;
- to treat any underlying infection (e.g. urinary tract infection, otitis media) which might have caused fever;
- to prevent further febrile convulsions.

Febrile convulsions in most children stop of their own accord, usually after 4–5 minutes. Short-lived febrile convulsions are not dangerous and do not cause brain damage. If a child convulses for more than 10 minutes then a doctor *must* be called immediately, or the child must be taken to the Accident and Emergency department of the nearest hospital. It is important to try and stop a convulsion, as there is a slight risk that prolonged febrile convulsions, lasting more than 30 minutes, may contribute to the later development of epilepsy (see p. 30). In order to stop a prolonged febrile convulsion, a doctor may give a medicine called diazepam (also called Valium or Stesolid), either by an injection into a vein or by a small tube inserted into the rectum, from which it is rapidly absorbed.

Some children who have had a first febrile convulsion will be admitted to hospital for observation and to find a cause of any underlying infection. Antibiotics may be given if an infection is found. A time in hospital may help to relieve parental anxiety. Interviews have revealed that the parents of at least half of the children who have their first febrile convulsion believe that their child is about to die, or has died. It is important to understand this concern and anxiety, to explain that this almost never happens, and reassure that children almost always make a full recovery following a febrile convulsion.

About one third of children will have a second or even third febrile convulsion. The risk of a child having a second or third febrile convulsion is greater if:

- the child is aged less than 12–15 months (and particularly if a girl);

- if the *first* febrile convulsion lasted more than 15–20 minutes or involved only one side of the body (i.e. was a complex febrile convulsion);

- if the parents or brother or sister has had febrile convulsions, or has epilepsy.

There are some simple measures which can be taken to prevent further or recurrent febrile seizures. These measures include (whenever a child has an infection and is showing a rise in temperature):

- undressing the child;

- sponging him or her with tepid (lukewarm) water, and

- giving regular paracetamol (Calpol) (every 3–4 hours) which brings down the temperature. It is not a good idea to use aspirin for this purpose in very young children, as this drug may bring on further problems in the liver.

There are certain situations in which a parent might anticipate that a child's temperature may well increase, and therefore that a febrile convulsion *may* occur. Such a situation might be after an immunization or vaccination (for example, the 'triple' vaccine, given three times in the first year of life, or the MMR (mumps, measles, rubella) vaccine given between 15 and 18 months of age). It is quite safe and sensible to give paracetamol at the time of vaccination and for 24–48 hours afterwards. With the MMR vaccine, there may be a very mild measles-like illness (with a high fever) 8–10 days after the vaccine has been given, and again, it would be wise to anticipate this and give paracetamol around that time.

In the past, anti-epileptic drugs were used to try and prevent further febrile convulsions from happening. It was shown that sodium valproate (Epilim) and phenytoin (Epanutin) were unsuccessful in preventing further febrile convulsions, and also did not alter the occurrence of convulsions without fever—that is, epileptic seizures. Although phenobarbitone has been shown to be effective in certain cases, this drug may cause significant side-effects in young children. In those few children who have repeated or long febrile convulsions, diazepam (Valium, Stesolid) may be given rectally, by parents after brief training. This medicine is used to prevent or stop the convulsion from lasting more than 30 minutes, but is only rarely necessary.

In a large prospective study of over 50 000 children carried out by the National Institute of Neurological and Communicative Disorders and Strokes in the USA, the incidence of febrile convulsions was 3.1 per cent, and the recurrence rate 32 per cent. By the time that the children had reached the age of seven years, more than one non-febrile seizure (that is, epilepsy) had developed in 0.5 per cent of those who had *never* had a febrile convulsion, and in four times as many—2 per cent—of those who *had* had a febrile convulsion. Children who had had prolonged or focal febrile convulsions, with evidence of pre-existing impaired development, were eight times more likely to develop epilepsy by the age of seven years than children with simple febrile convulsions, and 18 times more likely than children who had never had a febrile convulsion at all.

These figures show that one cannot deny the relation between some febrile convulsions (the complex and prolonged) and epilepsy. However, the parents of a child with one uncomplicated convulsion who has developed normally can be assured that the chances of subsequent epilepsy developing are very low—that the child has about 98 chances out of 100 of reaching the age of seven years without the occurrence of non-febrile seizures.

10 *The promise of the future*

The understanding and treatment of epilepsy has improved considerably over the past fifty years. Most of this improvement has resulted from basic scientific research into how and why epileptic seizures start, and from the development of safer and more effective anti-epileptic drugs by the pharmaceutical industry. However, there is still much work which needs to be carried out, not just to improve our understanding and knowledge, but to improve the quality of life of a child or man or woman with epilepsy.

It is unlikely that a single 'cure' for all epileptic seizures and epilepsies will be found, due to the fact that there are so many different causes and types of epilepsy. It is also very unlikely that epilepsies will ever be completely prevented from occurring in the first place. A proportion of the epilepsies are inherited. It is improbable that much can be done to prevent these epilepsies, and it may not be possible (or appropriate) to remove these abnormal genes by 'genetic engineering' techniques. However, improved medical care should reduce the numbers of patients who develop epilepsy after meningitis or encephalitis. Improved safety measures on the roads, in cars, and the wider use of cycle helmets and protective head gear on industrial sites should reduce the incidence of post-traumatic epilepsy. In developing countries, better obstetric care and public health measures to eradicate parasitic diseases, (particularly cysticercosis) and bacterial diseases (particularly tuberculosis and other causes of meningitis) will play a part.

New drugs

In the past, many new drugs were tested on their ability to stop experimental seizures in animals. This is what happened with drugs such as phenobarbitone, phenytoin, carbamazepine, and sodium valproate. Because such a drug's action is not just on stopping seizures, other effects, some adverse, are common. More recently through biochemical and neurological research, a number of chemicals (including neurotransmitters (p. 2)), have been identified which appear to have a crucial role in epilepsy. One of these, gamma aminobutyric acid (GABA), acts by inhibiting or stopping seizures. One new drug, vigabatrin, has been developed to increase the concentration of this substance within the brain, and so prevent seizures from happening. Other neurotransmitters called glutamate and aspartate can stimulate a seizure, or make a seizure more likely to happen. Lamotrigine is a new drug designed specifically to reduce the concentration of these substances in the brain and therefore prevent seizures. There are other drugs which are being assessed in a similar way, and which may become generally available in the next few years. Examples include gabapentin, oxcarbazepine, topirimate, remacemide, and zonisamide. It is to be hoped that such drugs 'tailor-made' to interfere with specific chemical processes will be associated with fewer side-effects, and will therefore be safer, and more acceptable to patients.

Surgery

It is likely that the surgical treatment of epilepsy will increase over the next decade. This is because scanning and EEG techniques will become more advanced, and more widely available, thereby enabling the identification of subtle abnormalities within the brain responsible for seizures, some of which will be capable of being removed surgically. It is likely that more specialist centres will become established to perform such surgery, and the operations will be undertaken at a younger age. However, as stated in Chapter 6, it will continue to be likely that only a relatively small number of patients will be suitable for surgical treatment.

Quality of life of children and people with epilepsy

Until comparatively recently, the emphasis of neurologists and pae-diatricians has been on obtaining complete control of epilepsy. The child or person's own feelings have not been taken into sufficient account, nor has the effect of epilepsy on aspects of their life such as choice of career, employment, social and leisure activities, and family life. The stigma which is associated with epilepsy, and the relatively poor medical understanding and management of epilepsy has contributed to patients with epilepsy experiencing a poor quality of life. This is now changing. Favourable factors are:

- an increased understanding about how epilepsy is caused;

- an increased medical awareness of the condition at all levels of undergraduate and postgraduate medical training;

- the development of more effective and safer drugs, and of surgical treatments leading to improved control of seizures;

- the development of clinics and facilities, both locally in general hospitals and nationally in major specialist centres;

- the appointment of specialist nurses in epilepsy whose role is to support and counsel patients of any age, and their families; and

- an expansion of local and national voluntary associations to provide advice and information to all patients and professionals who are involved with epilepsy.

The introduction of epilepsy clinics and specialist nurses in epilepsy are, in our view, as (if not more) important than the discovery of new anti-epileptic drugs in improving the quality of life of patients who have epilepsy.

Funding for research into epilepsy

Unfortunately, many of the above facilities are not yet available due to lack of funding, the relative lack of which also affects opportunities for research, and for attracting young researchers into the field. Epilepsy is, unfortunately, not regarded as important as many other clinical disorders when it comes to allocating funds for research. With the recent development of new anti-epileptic drugs, the pharmaceutical industry has provided generous support and sponsorship, particularly in areas of patient and professional education. Government and university departments and large charitable organizations are other important sources of funding for research and development.

Progress is likely to occur by the gradual accretion of new knowledge. There are journals, such as *Epilepsia, Epilepsy Research*, and *Seizure* devoted to publication of the results of the best research in epilepsy. There are also regular international meetings of those interested in epilepsy, so any real advance will be rapidly disseminated throughout the world.

The lot of those with epilepsy would be greatly improved, even if their seizures continued, if others—especially those involved with education and employers—showed greater understanding of their intermittent disability. The most probable benefit for the present generation of those with epilepsy is likely to result from such increased tolerance, rather than from any dramatic advances in treatment. Tolerance depends upon understanding the facts about epilepsy. We hope this book will help.

Appendix: International associations for those with epilepsy

National Epilepsy Association
PO Box 224
Parramatta NSW 2150   *Australia*
tel.no.: +61 2 891 6118
fax.no.: +61 2 891 6137

Elterninitiative für anafallskranke
Kinder
Stumpergasse 1/15
1060 Wien   *Austria*

Les Amis de la Ligue Nat.
Belge contre
l'Epilepsie
135 Avenue Albert
Brussels 1060   *Belgium*
tel.no.: +32 2 3443263

Epilepsy Canada
1470 Peelstreet, suite 745
Montreal, Quebec H3A 1T1 *Canada*
tel.no.: +1 514 845 7855
fax.no.: +1 514 845 7866

Ass. Liga c.l. Epilepsia de
Valparaiso
PO Box 705
Viña del Mar   *Chile*

Liga Colombiana contra la
Epilepsia
PO Box 057751
Bogota DC   *Colombia*
tel.no.: +57 1 2455717/2850788

Cuban Chapter of IBE
Zona Postal 4, Apartado
4248
C.Habana 10400   *Cuba*

Dansk Epilepsiforening
Dr. Sellsvej 28
DK 4293 Dianalund   *Denmark*
tel.no.: +45 58 26 44 66
fax.no.: +45 58 26 44 51

British Epilepsy Association
Anstey House
40 Hanover Square
Leeds LS3 1BE   *England*
tel.no.: +44 532 439393
fax.no.: +44 532 428804

Asox. de Padres de Niños con
Epilepsia
Casilla Postal 221
C Suc. 15
Quito   *Ecuador*

Epilepsialiitto
Kalevankatu 61
00180 Helsinki 18   *Finland*
tel.no.: +358 0 694 8433
fax.no.: +358 - 694 9927

A.I.S.P.A.C.E
11 Avenue Kennedy
F-59800 Lille   *France*
tel.no.: +33 20 92 65 33
fax.no.: +33 20 09 41 24

Deutsche Epilepsie Vereinigung
Sulzaer Str. 5
1000 Berlin 33   *Germany*
tel.no.: +49 30 826 6194
fax.no.: +49 30 826 7229

Greek National Assoc. against
Epilepsy
Aghia Sophia Children's
Hospital
Dept. of Neurology/
Neurophysiology
Athens 11527   *Greece*
tel.no.: +30 1 7771811
fax.no.: +30 1 7797649

Perpei
Jl. Jelita Utara no. 11
Rawamangun
Jakarta 13220   *Indonesia*
tel.no.: +62 21 797 0515
fax.no.: +62 21 797 0533

Indian Epilepsy Association
1, Old Veterinary Hospital Road
Basavanagudi
Bangalore 560 004   *India*
tel.no.: +91 812 6612778

Irish Epilepsy Association
249 Crumlin Road
Dublin 12   *Ireland*
tel.no.: +353 1 4557 500
fax.no.: +353 1 4557 013

Israel Epilepsy Association
PO Box 1598
Jerusalem   *Israel*
tel.no.:+ 972 2 371044

Associazione Italiana contro
l'Epilessia
Via Assarotti 44/4
16122 Genoa   *Italy*
tel.no.: +39 10 839 1767
fax.no.: +39 10 839 3822

The Japanese Epilepsy Association
5F Zenkokuzaidan Building 2-2-8
Nishiwaseda Shinjuku-KU
Tokyo 162   *Japan*
tel.no.: +81 3 202 5661
fax.no.: +81 3 202 7235

Korean Epilepsy Association
204-1 Yeonhi-dong, Seodaemun-ku
Seoul 120 – 112   *Korea*
tel.no.: +82 2 324 8400
fax.no.: +82 2 332 3728

Grupo Aceptacion de Epilepticos
Amsterdam 1928 # 19
Colonia Olimpica-Pedregal
Mexico 04710 D.F.   *Mexico*

Epilepsy Association of Scotland
48 Govan Road
Glasgow G5 1JI   *Scotland*
tel.no.: +44 41 427 4911
fax.no.: +44 41 427 7414

Epilepsie Vereniging Nederland
Hart. Nibbrigkade 71, flat 48
2597 XS Den Haag *The Netherlands*
tel.no.: + 31 30 66 01 44
fax.no.: + 31 30 66 05 10

Liga Proti Epilepsiji
CIPD, Njegoševa 4/11
61 000 Ljubljana   *Slovenia*
tel.no.: +38 6 61 482 006
fax.no.: +38 6 61 484 618

New Zealand Epilepsy Association
Inc.
PO Box 1074
Hamilton   *New Zealand*
tel.no.: +64 7 834 3556
fax.no.: +64 7 834 3553

South African National Epilepsy
League
PO Box 73
Observatory 7935   *South Africa*
tel.no.: +27 21 473014
fax.no.: +27 21 4485053

Norsk Epilepsiforbund
Storgt. 39
0192 Oslo   *Norway*
tel.no.: +47 22 206021
fax.no.: +47 22 115976

P.E.N.E.P.A.
Calle Escuelas Pia n. 89
08017 Barcelona   *Spain*
tel.no.: +34 3 3495400

Polish Epilepsy Association
Ul. Fabryczna 57 (XIp.pok.7)
15–482 Bialystok   *Poland*
tel.no.: +48 75 44 20

Epilepsy Association of Sri Lanka
10 Austin Place
Colombo 8   *Sri Lanka*
tel.no.: +94 1 696283

Liga Nacional Portuguesa c.l.
Epilepsia
Rua Sá da Bandeira 162-l o
4000 Porto   *Portugal*
tel.no.: +351 2 399 861
fax.no.: +351 2 302 515

Swedish Epilepsy Association
PO Box 9514
10274 Stockholm   *Sweden*
tel.no.: +46 8 669 4106
fax.no.: +46 8 669 1588

Schweizerische Liba gegen
Epilepsie
c/o Pro Infirmis
Postfach 129
8032 Zurich   *Switzerland*
tel.no.: +41 1 383 0531
fax.no.: +41 1 383 3049

Epilepsy Foundation of America
4351 Garden City Drive
Landover, Maryland 20785   *USA*
tel.no.: +1 301 459 3700
fax.no.: +1 301 577 2684

Epilepsy Support Foundation
P.O. Box A. 104
Avondale, Harare   *Zimbabwe*
tel.no.: +263 4 724 071

Montreal Neurological Institute
3801 University Street
Montreal Quebec H3A 2B4 *Canada*

Dianalund Epilepsy Hospital
DK 4293 Dianalund   *Denmark*
tel.no.: +45 3 564200

Liga Tung. de Control de la
Epilepsia
Cevallos 6-09 Y Montalvo,
officina 202
Segundo Piso Edificio Prof.
'Ambato'
Ambato   *Ecuador*

David Lewis Centre for Epilepsy
Near Alderley Edge
Cheshire, SK9 7UD   *England*
tel.no.: +44 565 872613
fax.no.: +44 565 872829

The National Society for Epilepsy
Chalfont Centre for Epilepsy
Chalfont St. Peter, Gerrards Cross
Buckinghamshire SL9 0RJ *England*
tel.no.: +44 494 873991
fax.no.: +44 494 871927

National Epilepsy Center
Shizuoka Higashi Hospital
886 Urushiyama,
Shizuoka 420   *Japan*
tel.no.: +81 542 45 5446
fax.no.: +81 542 46 1880

Dr. Hans Berger Kliniek
Postbus 90108
4800 RA Breda   *The Netherlands*
tel.no.: +31 76 608200/608465
fax.no.: +31 76 658954

Federatie voor Epilepsiebestrijding
PO Box 9587
3506 GN Utrecht *The Netherlands*
tel.no.: +31 30 660144
fax.no.: +31 30 660510

Institut voor Epilepsiebestrijding
Meer & Bosch/Cruquiushoeve
PO Box 21
2100 AA
Heemstede,   *The Netherlands*
tel.no.: +31 23 237237
fax.no.: +31 23 294324

Stichting Kempenhaeghe
Sterkselseweg 65
5591 VE Heeze   *The Netherlands*
tel.no.: +31 4907 79022
fax.no.: +31 4907 64924

Epilepsy Advisory Clinic
Z-438, Ratta Road
Rawalpindi   *Pakistan*
tel.no.: +92 51 550606

Quarrier's Homes
Bridge of Weir
Renfrewshire, PA11 3SA   *Scotland*

Epilepsy Care Centre, REEA
PO Box 41116, Craighall 2024
Johannesburg   *South Africa*
tel.no.: +27 11 788 4745
fax.no.: +27 11 788 4783

Epicentre, c/o Dominique Ūlkū
30B Chemin de la Colombe
1231 Conches   *Switzerland*
tel.no.: +41 22 346 43 53

Wales Epilepsy Association
Y pant teg Brynteg
Dolgellau, LL40 1RP
Gwynedd   *Wales*
tel.no.: +44 341 423339

Parke-Davis
Div. of Warner Lambert Company
201 Tabor Road
Morris Plains, N.Y. 07950   *USA*

Index

viral meningitis 37

West's syndrome 18, 32
  EEG 68
  prognosis 109
  treatment 105–6
women with epilepsy 124–5